Problem Periods

Problem Periods

Natural & Medical Solutions

Kaz Cooke
& Ruth Trickey

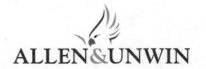

ALLEN&UNWIN

Thanks to Ge

Allen & Unwin
83 Alexander Street
Crows Nest NSW 2065
Australia
Phone: (61 2) 8425 0100
Fax: (61 2) 9906 2218
Email: info@allenandunwin.com
Web: www.allenandunwin.com

National Library of Australia
Cataloguing-in-Publication entry:

Cooke, Kaz, 1962– .
    Problem periods : natural & medical solutions.

    Includes index.
    1. Women – Health and hygiene. 2. Gynecology – Popular
    works. I. Trickey, Ruth, 1953– . II. Title.

618.1

Cover and text design by Dianna Wells Design
Set in 12/14 pt MrsEavesRoman by Bookhouse, Sydney
Printed in Australia by Griffin Press

10 9 8 7 6 5 4 3 2

Contents

hmmm

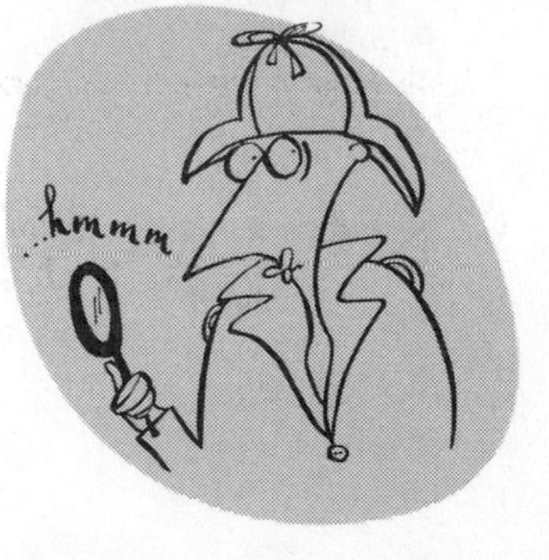

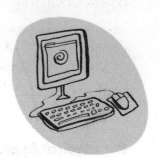

ABOUT THE AUTHORS

Ruth Trickey is a herbalist with a nursing and midwifery background. She specialises in herbal treatment of women's health problems. She runs the Melbourne Holistic Health Group in Melbourne, and treats many patients in conjunction with their doctors and surgeons. Ruth is the author of *Women, Hormones and The Menstrual Cycle*, and a frequent lecturer and guest speaker in Australia, New Zealand, Europe and North America.

Kaz Cooke is a cartoonist and author with a problem period past. She is the author of *Real Gorgeous: The truth about body and beauty*; *Up the Duff: The real guide to pregnancy*; *Living with Crazy Buttocks*; a children's book called *The Terrible Underpants* and the satirical 'Little Book of' series, encompassing *Stress, Dumb Feng Shui, Household Madness, Beauty*, and *Diet and Exercise*. www.kazcooke.com

Most of the information in this book is edited and updated from the text of *Women's Trouble: Natural and Medical Solutions*, by the same authors, also published by Allen & Unwin. A full list of acknowledgements and footnotes is published in *Women's Trouble*. Also in this series of small books on women's health: *Menopause* and *Endometriosis*.

All advice given in this book is general and not intended to be used instead of professional medical advice. Any of the advice herein should be undertaken only after consultation with your doctor and natural therapies practitioner. Each person in your advice team must be aware of all drugs, herbs and other treatments you are undergoing. It is not safe to self-diagnose, or self-prescribe with either herbs or drugs. Individual and tailored treatments can only be obtained from your own practitioners.

Intro

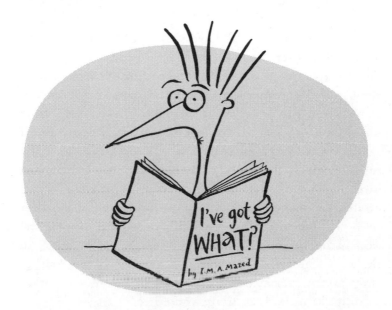

THE MODERN PERIOD

Menstruation, Fred, on the rag, periods, a visit from a friend, women's trouble, having the painters in — call it whatever you like. You're going to see a lot of it.

These days we start getting our periods at a younger age, eat better, use contraception, and live longer — so we have heaps more periods than women in the past. The 'average' Australian woman, let's call her Sheila, can expect to get her first period at about 12 years old, and then get pregnant between 25 and 35. Then she'll have two or three pregnancies about two years apart, breastfeeding for six to nine months each time. Sheila will go on having periods until she's about 50, when she hits menopause, gets a surge of new powerful feelings and decides to take over Microsoft.

A modern woman will have a total of between 360 and 400 periods over about 30 years. If you add it all together, we can expect to 'bleed' for a total of three years in a lifetime, about ten times more often than our ancestors. But don't yearn for yesteryear too much. "Ere, Nell. Fank Gawd we don't 'ave to 'ave lots of periods. I've got enuff to do wot with 17 kids darn wiv Black Death and the 'usband off at the bloody Crusades again.' In the past women got their first period at 14 or 15, started having endless pregnancies straightaway and died decades earlier than the current life expectancy of a non-Aboriginal woman in Australia. Without contraception or much in the way of independence, women were likely to be either pregnant or breastfeeding all the time, having an average of only 40 periods in their whole life.

Diet, lifestyle and stress can all easily affect the timing of your period and whether you'll have any pain. This has become less obvious since we've been able to drop a painkiller or go on the Pill as soon as there was a problem. But these days more people are interested in the delicacy of the menstrual cycle, and its dependency on nutrition and general health. Many of us would rather control or treat our period problems with commonsense and natural remedies before resorting to drugs. And most of us now want to know what's happening to our bodies.

The best way to start is by dealing quickly with any

deviations from your own, normal period pattern. This book is designed to explain what's normal, what's abnormal, how to recognise warning signs and be on the way to a diagnosis, and the best ways to approach treatment for five of the most common problems related to periods.

First up, it's important to recognise that periods are normal and healthy.

It's only relatively recently that some people have been able to come to terms with the perfectly normal fact of periods. Others are stuck back in the Black Death era when it comes to their attitudes to the strangely named issue of 'feminine hygiene'. ('That ad for unmentionables is on the telly again, Beryl. I'm going down the shed.')

What Is a Normal Period?

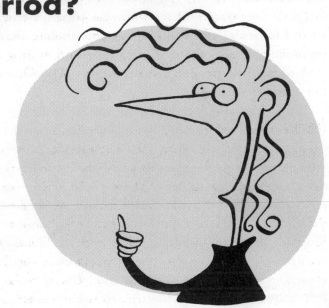

A period is the regular shedding of the endometrium — the lining of the uterus — once every month for most of us. It looks like blood, and we call it blood, but it's made up of other tissues and secretions as well as blood, from the inside of the uterus.

HOW YOUR PERIOD WORKS

Counting the days

The first bleeding day of a proper period is counted as Day One of your menstrual cycle. Premenstrual spotting,

 4

or 'false alarms' are not counted as part of a proper period. From the first day of the period to ovulation is the follicular (egg-making) phase, usually about 14 days long. (So technically, the menstrual phase is contained in the follicular phase.) The day you ovulate the luteal phase begins, also about 14 days long and ending at the start of the next proper period, which is Day One of the next cycle.

The hormonal menstrual cycle

All the time, inside us, we produce varying levels of the sex hormones which set up a regular menstrual cycle. You seething sexual being, you. There's a lot going on, with various departments at work. The main departments are the endocrine glands found in the hypothalamus and the pituitary in the brain, and in the ovaries. These are responsible for hormone production and cycle regulation. (Sometimes this inter-departmental hormone-making action is called the 'hypothalamic-pituitary-ovarian unit' or the 'hormonal axis', or 'that thingy with the really long name'.)

The endocrine glands work together, sending messages by hormones and setting up a 'feedback loop' which means that as one hormone level falls it triggers another one to start, and when that one starts it triggers another one to fall, so the cycle continues month after month.

The feedback loop works something like this: during the cycle, the hypothalamus produces gonadotrophin releasing hormone (GnRH), which reminds the pituitary to produce luteinising hormone (LH) and follicle stimulating hormone (FSH), which signals the ovaries to release oestrogen and progesterone, which are recognised by the hypothalamus, which then produces GnRH again … so it all rolls around, the same sequence, over and over and over, like the plot of a Mills and Boon novel.

The follicular phase

All the hormones have special jobs to do in the loop. For example, the FSH starts the eggs growing in an ovary — at that stage the egg is called a follicle. Between 10 and 20 follicles may begin to develop, but only one of these will become dominant and mature completely to become an ovum, or egg. The others fade away and by the time of ovulation the mature follicle is the only one remaining, ready to go.

While the follicles are developing, they produce more and more oestrogen which stimulates the endometrium, the cells lining the womb, to grow like mad, known as proliferation. (The proliferative phase and the follicular phase are interchangeable terms.) When the egg is maturing, so is the uterine lining. The length of this phase is variable, but it starts immediately after a period. Oestrogen levels continue to increase while the egg develops. Eventually, the increasing levels trigger a big effort from the feedback loop to pump out the right hormone levels which trigger the release of the egg. There's your ovulation.

The luteal phase

Ovulation is followed by the luteal phase. This stage of the cycle takes its name from the corpus luteum, the remnant of the follicle where the egg developed. The corpus luteum, influenced by the feedback loop, now starts to secrete increasing quantities of progesterone and, after an initial drop, fairly constant levels of oestrogen.

This luteal phase corresponds with the secretory phase of the endometrium. Progesterone and oestrogen act together on the endometrium causing it to become a 'secretory' tissue building up a thick glycogen-rich tissue, where a fertilised egg could embed and develop.

If the egg isn't fertilised, the corpus luteum fades away after its two-week work of producing oestrogen and progesterone, and the hormone output falls. A combination of factors including hormone levels, blood and tissue changes and prostaglandins activity causes the endometrium, which has by now reached its maximum thickness of about 8 millimetres, to degenerate. Uterine contractions help it on its way down the hatch as a period. Welcome to the menstrual phase.

A 'NORMAL' PERIOD

Right. A normal period is when a girl called Susan in a textbook has a period exactly every 28 days, for precisely five days, after which it stops like a tap going off. And it is important to note that Susan continues to ride her pony, Fluffball, throughout the entire ordeal. If your name isn't Susan and you don't have a pony, your period is probably abnormal. Or maybe we should think about it another way.

'Normal' is a strange word to use for periods, because the range of possibilities is so wide and there are so many exceptions to the rule that are just as 'normal'. It's probably easier to say what's abnormal. So let's just say we'll look at the most usual kinds of periods you can have.

Susan's is known as the 'textbook period', because it appears in every boring old textbook and if textbooks had periods it would be exactly like this: a menstrual cycle is 28 days long with a period lasting three to five days. The luteal phase (between ovulation and the start of the period) will be 14 days long to the second, and the follicular phase (from the start of the period to ovulation) will also miraculously be exactly 14 days long.

Needless to say lots of us don't have this exact pattern — so it makes more sense to talk about a normal range of possible times for each event.

These are the big ticket factors: how regular the cycle is; how long the whole cycle goes for; how long the period bleeding lasts; the amount of pain; and the colour and consistency of the blood.

A regular cycle

A regular cycle depends on ovulation, and on the hormone balance. Both can affect each other: not ovulating changes hormone levels, and a hormonal imbalance may interfere with the set-up for ovulation.

The most variable part of the cycle is usually the follicular phase, the time when the egg is developing, ready for ovulation. As teenagers, many of us ovulate erratically for months, when our periods first start, as our body tries to establish regular 'communication' between the hormones to get the feedback loop going. Just imagine bits of the hormonal feedback loop as a scattered gang with walkie-talkies: 'Hello ovaries, come in please.' 'This is the hypothalamus.' 'Get off the line, I'm trying to talk to the ovaries. Over.' 'Roger. Am I supposed to be doing anything?' 'What? Who's Roger?' 'Who are you?' 'Oestrogen, I think.' 'Does anybody know what time to get follicular?' and so on.

Eventually they'll all get their act together, but at this age it's also easier for stress or change to confuse the hormonal interplay and interrupt the regularity of the cycle. Erratic ovulation will make for an 'earlier' or 'later' period.

As you approach menopause you might also have an irregular cycle because there are fewer eggs being made and because the hormonal feedback loop slows down, so ovulation isn't triggered so regularly, or in the end, at all. Stress is also more likely to get in the way of a regular cycle around the time of the menopause.

Missing a period

Pregnancy is the most usual cause of a missed period, and to mutter the obvious, much more likely if you've not used contraception. Pregnancy tests which measure hormone levels in your wee are available from chemists or doctors, and will give an accurate result within days of becoming pregnant, even before the next period would be due. Blood tests can be accurate as early as ten days after fertilisation, but wait until 14 days to be absolutely sure of not getting a false negative result.

Don't worry too much if you miss a period, and you know you're not pregnant. A missed period is often just a hormonal or ovulatory 'hiccup' caused by stress (either horrible or fun) or by illness. The hormonal axis, or as we now know it, the incredibly complicated whole hormonal thingy, is very delicate and can be easily confused, temporarily. You'll usually re-establish a normal pattern once the episode is over — unless you get so stressed at missing a period you make your body do it all over again! You may well completely stop periods when travelling and for some time after you come home. Quick weight loss due to illness, poor diet or irregular patterns of sleep and activity common amongst travellers may be the real culprits. If you're travelling or otherwise stressed, try to maintain a regular lifestyle and diet pattern and you'll avoid associated problems like loss of bone density.

And don't assume that if you have irregular periods you can't get pregnant and don't need contraception. Missing a period or even a series of periods does not necessarily imply infertility. Ovulation can spontaneously sneak up on you at any time. Of course, not expecting a period, you mightn't realise you're pregnant for a few months. It then might be too late to safely have a pregnancy termination; or those few too many drinks and cigarettes might have harmed the developing embryo.

Contraception options can be explored at a Family Planning Clinic or local doctor. May we put in a good word for the humble and particularly splendid condom — because when used properly (i.e. 'No, Darryl I don't think it goes on your ear. Read the instructions, pie-face.') it's the only contraception to protect against sexually transmitted diseases. (And, just to make it all a bit more eeky, many sexually transmitted diseases have female infertility as a possible side effect.) Missing a period for more than six months is a recognised condition needing investigation, and we'll get on to that later.

The length of the cycle
Most menstrual cycles are between 21 and 35 days long. You might have cycles that are regularly longer or shorter than this pattern but if you're physically well, eating properly, full of beans and raring to party, at a reasonable weight for your height; and have a problem-free period, your cycle is normal for you.

Very short cycles can be caused by erratic ovulation. (They can be mistaken for mid-cycle bleeding.) And very long cycles can be a problem if you're trying to get pregnant. You might even have regularly irregular cycles. This is usually a sign of erratic ovulatory patterns, which, although not 'normal', isn't a serious health problem. You might, however, develop dysfunctional uterine bleeding (DUB) – one of the topics of this book – which does need treating in most cases.

You should see a health care practitioner if you have very short or very long cycles and you also have signs of ill health, or if you start having deviations from your own usual cycle length.

The length of the period
Between three and five days of bleeding is the accepted length of a normal period. Periods that last for fewer days may be related to a number of conditions including thyroid disorders, anaemia and low body weight.

Longer periods may be an indication of hormonal imbalance, in particular that you're not ovulating, a process dependent upon normal hormone interactions. Very long periods can also be a sign of disorders and some serious gynaecological conditions.

The length of a period does not include any days you have pre- or post-period spotting. Spotting near the time of a period can be an indication of serious problems and may need to be investigated; and any spotting between periods must be reported to a doctor as soon as possible.

The amount of blood

Basically, if you need to change a pad or tampon more often than after two hours because it is totally soaked with blood (not just because you like to change that often), and you need to do this all day or for longer during your period, that's heavy bleeding. If your pad has just a line of blood down the middle or your tampon has less than the top third absorbed with blood, and you only 'bleed' for a day, that's a very light period.

Even if your pad or tampon doesn't get fully 'used' they should be changed at least every four hours or so. Keeping a record in your diary or on a menstrual symptom calendar is a helpful way of keeping track of bleeding for you and also to report to your health care practitioner.

A common cause of heavy bleeding is fibroids, while light and erratic bleeding is often seen in association with polycystic ovarian syndrome (PCOS), which is discussed in detail later in the book. Many other conditions that can cause heavy, light, or erratic periods are explored in the hormones and usual suspects section. It's worth noting that DUB (dysfunctional uterine bleeding, page 106) can cause a range of problem periods.

Period pain

Unless you move in long-distance swimming circles, any mysterious mention of 'the cramps' is always assumed to be about period pain. So many of us get period pain that it could be called usual — but that doesn't make it normal. The pain response is a survival mechanism indicating that something has gone wrong. Here's the basic rule of judging period pain: is it bad enough that you want to do something about it?

Period pain usually only happens in a cycle that you have ovulated in, and period pain often only starts in earnest about two years after the first-ever period, when ovulation has become regular. That's why an occasional period can be surprisingly pain-free — maybe you didn't ovulate in that cycle. There's a whole section on period pain later on.

An odd period

Most of us will have at least one 'odd' period in our lives; some will have lots. The cycle may be unusual, the flow different from normal; pain may be new or different; or the colour and consistency of the blood might change.

Here's what you need to ask about a strange period:
· Is it possible you're pregnant?
· Are there other signs of ill health?
· Has there been a stressful episode (either fun or diffi-
  cult)?

If the answer to either of the first two questions is yes,

get thee to a doctor. If the third option is a possibility, have a cup of tea and a good lie down; in other words, relax, wait for another cycle and see what happens.

Period symptoms diary

On the facing page is a detailed menstrual symptom diary you can photocopy and use to chart your period's regularity and all the symptoms associated with it. It will help you work out if you have PMS, and what type of PMS, for example. (See the PMS section for the whole deal on this subject.) It will also be indispensable in helping your health practitioner to diagnose a problem. Keep a photocopy for yourself.

YOUR HORMONES – WHAT THEY ARE AND WHAT THEY DO

Feel free to skip this whole section if you don't want to get down into the nitty gritty of your complicated little critters like hormones and prostaglandins. Don't mind us. We've just spent months researching it and trying to make it as simple as possible. And none of your girly bits would do their thing without the hormones. But you don't really need to read it, unless you really want to know how your body works, or you have a hormone problem. On the other hand, it will help you better understand a whole lot of problems – ranging from period cramps caused by prostaglandins imbalance, to stopped periods that can be kick-started again by fiddling with hormone levels.

PERIOD SYMPTOMS DIARY: Record the relevant coded number to describe your bleeding and symptoms.

BLEEDING: 0—none 1—slight 2—moderate 3—heavy 4—heavy and clots
SYMPTOMS: 0—none 1—mild; does not interfere with activities 2—moderate; interferes with activities 3—severe; disabling; unable to function

Day of cycle	1	2	3	4	5	6	7	8	9	10	11	12	13	14	15	16	17	18	19	20	21	22	23	24	25	26	27	28	29	30	31	32	33	34	35	36
DATE																																				
BLEEDING																																				
PMS-A SYMPTOMS:																																				
Nervous tension																																				
Mood swings																																				
Irritability																																				
Anxiety																																				
PMS-H SYMPTOMS:																																				
Weight gain																																				
Swelling of extremities																																				
Breast tenderness																																				
Abdominal bloating																																				
PMS-C SYMPTOMS:																																				
Headache																																				
Craving for sweets																																				
Increased appetite																																				
Heart pounding																																				
Fatigue																																				
Dizziness or faintness																																				
PMS-D SYMPTOMS:																																				
Depression																																				
Forgetfulness																																				
Crying																																				
Confusion																																				
Insomnia																																				
PMS-P SYMPTOMS:																																				
Pain																																				
Cramps																																				
Backache																																				
General aches/pain																																				

You can photocopy this diary to use indefinitely.

Meet your hormones

All month long, a whole bunch of hormones get together and do a funky hormone dance to make the menstrual cycle work. Alright, forget the dance metaphor. This is complicated enough already — let's get scientific. The hormones that are the main players are all 'steroid hormones'. The steroids are all made by the body using the chemical building block of cholesterol. They are the androgens (pronounced and-roe-jens), oestrogens (east-roe-jens) and progesterones (pr-oh-jest-er-owns).

Some hormones start off as one kind, and are then made into a series of other hormones so they can perform the right tasks to make the whole menstrual cycle pump along.

For example, one hormone starts out called preg-nenolone, is then changed by the body into progesterone, then to testosterone and finally into one of the oestro-gens, called oestradiol. At each step, the hormone will have a special job to do. At the end of the line each hormone is changed into a different form, into another type of hormone, or broken down to be excreted from the body.

Before its life is finished, each hormone will have an intricate part to play in the 'feedback loop' which runs the menstrual cycle month after month. But the really big players are progesterone and oestrogen.

For everything to go smoothly, the hormones must remain in some sort of balance with each other, and like actors they all must make their entrance and exit at the right time. (Great, now we've got a theatre metaphor.)

We're going to briefly look at how each hormone is involved. You wouldn't believe all the stuff your body gets up to when you're not looking.

The Stage Manager hormones

The hypothalamus, a gland at the base of the brain, produces a number of stage manager hormones which send messages to tell other hormones when to do their stuff in the cycle. Or, these stage manager hormones block the other hormones until their cue to come on.

Gonadotrophin releasing hormone (GnRH)

The hypothalamus sends messages to the nearby pituitary gland in the form of intermittent pulses of GnRH every 60 to 90 minutes. The pulsing of GnRH increases mid-cycle and around the period, and reminds the pituitary when it's time to pump out extra follicle stimulating hormone (FSH) and luteinising hormone (LH).

Dopamine

If you are not breastfeeding, the hypothalamus also releases sufficient quantities of a hormone called dopamine to control the production of prolactin, the hormone responsible for producing breast milk.

The Director hormones

The pituitary gland produces gonadotrophins, bossy hormones which tell ovaries what to do. In other words, these are the director hormones who tell the other hormones when to play their roles.

Luteinising hormone (LH)

Low levels of oestrogen trigger the slow rise of LH levels during the follicular, egg-making phase of the cycle. Just before mid-cycle, a dramatic surge in oestrogen, LH, and FSH causes ovulation. The LH stimulates the ovaries to make more oestrogen and progesterone. In the luteal, post-ovulation phase, the increasing progesterone levels signal the pituitary gland to hold back on the LH. Further push-me pull-you stuff between the hormones finally triggers the period.

Follicle stimulating hormone (FSH)

Follicle stimulating hormone (FSH) does exactly what its name suggests — stimulates the growth and development of the ovarian follicle — the bit which houses an egg. Levels of FSH increase in the follicular, egg-making phase of the cycle, which reminds the follicle cells to pump out some more oestrogen. This is all part of the feedback loop — the initial rise in oestrogen triggers the release of GnRH and a surge of FSH. A few hours later, when oestrogen levels are even higher, FSH production is turned off. Just before a period, oestrogen levels fall, which reminds the hypothalamus to send out a hormonal message of GnRH to the pituitary and get it to start releasing FSH again.

Prolactin

Prolactin, produced by the pituitary gland, is the hormone responsible for breast milk, and for making your breasts bigger during pregnancy. Non-pregnant women have low levels of prolactin which normally increase slightly at night, with stress, and during the luteal phase of the menstrual cycle.

The Star Actor hormones

The ovaries and the adrenal glands above the kidneys make the steroid hormones oestrogen, androgen and progesterone. These 'actor' hormones do most of the heavy work. As girly hormones go, they are the stars.

Oestrogen

Oestrogen is the big-time player — in fact there are three main oestrogens — oestradiol (pronounced east-rar-dye-al), oestrone (east-rone) and oestriol (east-ree-ol). When people talk about oestrogen or oestrogen levels, they usually mean the cumulative effect of these three in the body, even though it sounds like there's one oestrogen diva going at it all alone.

Some of the effects of oestrogen are most obvious during puberty. Oestrogen gives you a proper girly stomach and hips and breasts. It stimulates the growth of the uterine muscle and endometrium. All through life, oestrogen helps to maintain skin structure, blood vessels, and bone strength.

One of the most important functions of oestrogen is to stimulate an increase in the number of cells (proliferation) where there are oestrogen receptors, for example, in the endometrium.

The lifespan of the oestrogens

Every month after the period, the ovaries start to secrete active oestrogen called oestradiol. Some of the oestradiol is converted into a weaker oestrogen called oestrone, and then both oestradiol and oestrone go on a trip together in the bloodstream, travelling to exotic lands ... sorry. They travel to oestrogen-sensitive cells to stimulate cell growth. The ovaries pump out the most oestrogen after ovulation, and cut back just before the period.

Meanwhile, the body makes a second source of oestrone from androgen hormones. This process, using an enzyme, is referred to as 'peripheral conversion' or 'aromatisation'. Aromatisation happens in the hair follicles, the skin, the brain, bone and bone marrow, muscle and fatty tissue. About 25 per cent of the conversion goes on in the muscle and 10–15 per cent in the fat. (After the menopause, we make almost all our oestrogen from aromatisation, as our ovaries 'retire'.)

The rest of us manufacture most of our oestrogen, in the form of oestradiol, in the ovaries. We also make some oestrone from androgens, mostly by the aromatisation in our fatty tissues. If you're thinner than your body should be, you mightn't get enough of this important secondary source of oestrogen and could develop menopausal symptoms like hot flushes and vaginal dryness; or may stop ovulating and having periods. If you're obese, you may be making too much oestrogen and be at risk of conditions linked to too much oestrogen, including breast cancer and endometrial cancer.

Eventually, all the different oestrogens are carried to the liver. There they change into different forms which are less active, and are sent to the intestine. Once in the intestine, some of the oestrogen will be excreted from the bowel and some will be recycled back into the bloodstream.

All of the oestrogen circulating in the blood will eventually pass through the kidneys where it is excreted in the urine as the very weak oestrogen called oestriol. This forms the basis of some pregnancy tests and can be used to determine the health of the placenta during pregnancy. Although it contributes to the oestrogen pool, oestriol is about 80 times less potent than oestradiol.

The 'oestrogen pool'
Sounds like a rather good name for a sexy nightclub, but it refers to the range of oestrogens available for use by the body. There are many factors that cause oestrogenic effects which can come from outside the body. These include the phyto-oestrogens produced in plants, which are good for you; and the much more dangerous 'environmental oestrogens', which are consumed as hormones added to foods or as contaminants of foods, such as pesticides. All of these different types of 'oestrogens' can have oestrogen-like activities in the body.

An oestrogenic effect is caused by any substance which has the ability to connect to an oestrogen receptor site. It has to be said, quite frankly, that oestrogen receptor sites are pretty stupid, and will often accept any substance which has a molecular similarity to the oestrogen produced in the body, even if it's a chemical pesticide.

The receptor sites can be monopolised by oestrogen-like substances from plants which don't have a very strong oestrogenic effect. The substances have, in a way, taken most of the oestrogen parking spaces. The stronger oestrogens, made in the body, can't get as many parks, so they can't go to work and do their stuff.

In this way the body can be exposed to a weaker combination of oestrogens. Before menopause, this can help protect against the disorders linked to having too much oestrogen. After menopause, when you're not making so much oestrogen in your own body because your ovaries have 'retired', plant oestrogens or oestrogenic herbs can help fill all the empty parking spaces and help boost your depleted 'oestrogen pool'.

The available information on the nastier 'environmental oestrogens' is less clear. There are a whole heap of chemicals which may work in combination to cause strong oestrogenic effects. These include the pesticides such as endosulphan, toxaphene, dieldrin, chlordecone, DDT and DDE; the polychlorinated biphenols (PCBs) found in a range of products such as hydraulic fluid, neon tubes and plastics such as nonylphenol released from modified polystyrene; bisphenol-A, a plastic found in the 'lacquer' used to coat food cans; and other plastics used as a substitute for mercury-based amalgam fillings.

The real health implications of these chemicals are unknown. Research is continuing to see if there is a link between exposure to insecticides and cancer development. High levels of DDT have, however, been found in fibroid tissue, and there are concerns that these chemicals may affect male fertility and sexual development, and increase cancer risk.

Exposure to chemicals will have varying effects on different people depending on how long they were exposed, which chemicals, and their body's elimination systems. And even though some of these products have only a weak oestrogenic effect, they must be suspected of some harm because many are poisons designed to kill plant or insect life. Suffice to say it's probably safer to stay away from DDT sandwiches and try to minimise the use of chemicals in your body, your home and your local area.

Progesterone

Progesterone, the other big star of girly hormones, is the building block starter for many of the other steroid hormones. So it plays an important role not only in periods and reproduction, but also in a number of other jobs in the body.

It stimulates changes in organs with progesterone-sensitive tissue. In the uterus, progesterone stimulates the endometrium so that it can support a developing embryo. If the egg is not fertilised, the level of progesterone falls, the endometrial tissue disintegrates and is shed as a period.

Progesterone initiates glandular changes in breast tissue so that the breast is capable of giving milk. It also keeps the normal female levels of androgen (blokey) hormones in check. Once progesterone production slows or stops, like after menopause, androgen levels increase. This may account for hair falling out of the head but mysteriously turning up on the chin when some of us get older. Progesterone has other actions that include improved fat metabolism, an increase in bone density, good moods, and a natural diuretic (fluid loss) effect. It also helps to prevent both cancerous and benign breast changes by counterbalancing the effects of oestrogen in the breast, and has the same protective and counterbalancing effect on the endometrium.

Progesterone is also the building block of the hormones called corticosteroids which maintain stable blood sugar levels, reduce inflammation and help the body fight the effects of stress.

The lifespan of a progesterone

Progesterone is produced by the corpus luteum — the remnant egg sac — in the ovaries. Small amounts are also secreted by the adrenal glands. The body changes cholesterol into pregnenolone and then to progesterone. The progesterone might then be converted into any one of the other steroid hormones including oestradiol, oestrone, testosterone or cortisone.

Progesterone circulates in the blood and interacts with cell receptors, but eventually it will pass through the liver where it is 'turned off' and excreted into the bile and urine.

Androgens

Androgens are blokey hormones, found naturally in both men and women. When androgen levels are too high, such as in polycystic ovarian syndrome (PCOS), it can interfere with the menstrual cycle and gynaecological functions. It can also cause more hairiness, a deeper voice, and a more 'male' body shape, with smaller breasts and a larger waist.

The star of the blokey hormones is testosterone. You might be surprised to know that we've got some too.

Testosterone is the strongest and most abundant androgen found in the blood of normal women. A quarter of it is made in the ovaries, a quarter in the adrenal glands and half is made in the body by converting other hormones. In muscle, testosterone acts directly on the androgen receptors to produce growth-promoting ('anabolic') effects.

The carrier proteins

Most of the steroid hormones circulate in the blood transported by proteins (albumins and globulins). Each hormone appears to have a specific binding globulin or carrier protein which is responsible for its transport. When hormones are bound to the globulins, they can't interact as easily with target tissues as when they are floating 'free' in the plasma. For example, if a blokey androgen hormone isn't bound to carrier proteins it's more likely to be surging around in your blood giving you a hairy chin and other problems. So it's important to keep a good balance of carrier proteins.

Meet your prostaglandins

To work properly, ovulation, periods and childbirth all depend on the hormones to behave themselves. It is not so well known that they also rely on some complicated, hormone-like substances called prostaglandins to behave themselves as well.

Prostaglandins are made by the body to control heaps of different functions, for example, bleeding, clotting, anti-inflammatory action and muscle spasms. This makes them big players in the menstrual cycle, what with all that

25

experience in stopping and starting bleeding and controlling crampy things. Some prostaglandins might become too dominant in cases of infection, inflammation, allergy, hormone variations or poor diet. These imbalances may be temporary, or continue indefinitely, and are believed to be causes of period pain, heavy periods, PMS and endometriosis. (All of these problems have their own sections in this book, except for endo, which you can find out about in the sister book to this one, *Endometriosis*.)

It may help to think of prostaglandins as a large family of hormone-like substances which perform many functions throughout the body.

The prostaglandin family is really a sub-group of an extended family of microscopic substances found in most tissues called the eicosanoids (I-ko-san-oids). In the eicosanoid extended family, there are two clans — the large and well-known family called the prostaglandins, and a smaller branch of rellies called the leukotrienes. The prostaglandin family is itself made up of even smaller families, like nuclear families in an extended clan. These families include the prostacyclins and the thromboxanes as well as a group of individual prostaglandins. Each of the members of the extended family has a broad role to play: the prostaglandins influence blood clotting, the activity of muscles and the inflammatory responses throughout the body; the thromboxanes are involved with blood clotting and blood vessel activity; and the leukotrienes are regulators of inflammatory and allergic reactions. Whenever you bleed, get a scab, throw up or have a muscle spasm, there's a prostaglandin working overtime.

Within each of the thromboxane, prostaglandins and leukotriene families, each of the members has its own more detailed role. As with all families, some of the members tend to be nuisances, others are more useful. Just as some rellies are liable to go off the deep-end at any given time (especially Christmas), some of the rellies in the prostaglandin family can go a bit feral from time to time. And then there are the distant rellies — some of whom can be unreliable. For example, one of the leukotrienes will start some of the processes of inflammation, and another one, either a close or distant clan relative, will have the role of calming everything down.

The prostaglandins do various conflicting jobs in the menstrual cycle, so they need to be in balance. One type of prostaglandin stops platelets from clumping together and dilates blood vessels, which causes heavier period bleeding. Another prostaglandin strongly increases muscle contraction, but in the Fallopian tube, it causes relaxation. Another one is always complaining that the young people of today get it too good. Sorry, that's one of *my* relatives.

Rogue prostaglandins can be responsible for the crampy type of period pain, because some prostaglandins cause blood vessels in the endometrium to constrict and cause muscle spasm. When some are too dominant, it can cause period pain from the cramping muscle. And in general, leukotrienes stimulate uterus contractions, so when some of these leukotrienes go into overdrive, the contractions cause crampy period pain. One type of leukotriene attracts white cells to inflamed tissues and is found in high levels when women have endometriosis. It may also be involved in breast cancer.

Balancing the prostaglandins

The medical approach
In some cases of period pain, prostaglandins-inhibiting drugs will be prescribed. These are fully explained under Drugs in The Medical Approach chapter.

Natural therapies & self care
The body uses Omega-3 fatty acids and Omega-6 fatty acids to make leukotrienes, thromboxanes, and prostaglandins. The fatty acids that can treat conditions caused by an imbalance of prostaglandins are found in certain foods and should be regularly included in the diet. For the best healthy effects, you need to eat more essential fatty acids and less of the 'bad oils' which interfere with them. (Essential fatty acids, and what foods they're in, are explained under Bad Fats and Good Fats, number 8 of the 20 Good-Eating Hints in the Self Care chapter.) If you want to have balanced prostaglandins, it's essential that you read and follow it.

When Things Go Wrong

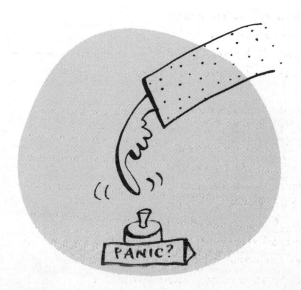

How will you know if something is abnormal? Well, if your horoscope says you are going to be eaten alive by a giant squid on Thursday, politicians seem honestly caring, you get to work and find that you've been replaced by a robot run on beetroot juice and Hollywood actually casts a leading actress who weighs more than a Mintie, there'll be an inkling that things are a wee bit strange.

On the subject of periods and related problems, if anything on the following list applies to you, then skedaddle off to a doctor for diagnosis. When you have a diagnosis, you can read the relevant bits in this book, and get treatment from a doctor and/or natural therapist.

WHEN TO SEE A DOCTOR

- There's no sign of the first period by 17 years old.
- Your period has stopped for more than a couple of months.
- There's a sudden change or series of changes in your menstrual cycle. For example you used to be regular as clockwork and now it's all over the shop, or you used to have a really light period and now you're wondering if you should buy tampons in bulk (an abnormally heavy period means suddenly needing to change pads or tampons every two hours) or any new and unusual pain related to the period.
- There's excessive pain during or before each period. (Excessive pain means the level of the pain interferes with or restricts your life — for example, you have to lie down with a hot-water bottle calling for Milo instead of going dancing.)
- If you're having abnormally long periods — which means longer than seven days if you don't usually bleed for that long.
- You bleed between each period even if it is very light.
- You have a yellowish or smelly vaginal discharge, or any vaginal itch or soreness.

The Usual Suspects

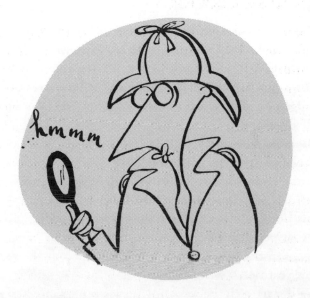

Heaps of different things can affect your period and the functions of the hormonal cycle: being stressed, being underweight, dieting, fasting, the amount of exercise you do and various drugs of the prescribed and not-so prescribed sort. If things are going wrong you might like to investigate the obvious possibilities first. These 'usual suspects' can be a lot easier to fix than the other diseases and disorders that can cause problems with your period. The most usual outcome of these 'suspects' is that they cause a change to the normal ebb and flow of your hormones, leading to a variety of hormonal imbalances.

Understanding how the 'usual suspects' affect hormonal imbalance won't stop you from getting any of the problems described in this book. For instance, some types of hormonal imbalances are inherited, such as those associated with PCOS, but even then, diet and lifestyle can have an impact on the severity of the complaint. Other types of hormonal problems, such as dysfunctional uterine bleeding (DUB), will have a greater tendency to occur when women approach menopause but how stressed you are might be the factor that determines whether or not it will develop.

Diet, exercise and stress also influence the severity and frequency of period pain and PMS. Sometimes, though we don't know why, some women develop fibroids. And sometimes why they've developed any of the complaints in this book is a complete mystery. So knowing how the 'usual suspects' affect hormones might not be much use to you. On the other hand, it might just offer the explanation you need.

We'll start with the ways hormones can be affected first and then look at each of the usual suspects in turn.

UNBALANCED HORMONES

Any hormone imbalance will have an effect on health. Hormone levels can be too high, be around for too long, or they can reach levels that are too high or too low in relation to other hormones. Women with endometriosis and fibroids, for example, are thought to have too much exposure to oestrogen for too long. If you have PMS you may have low levels of progesterone in relation to your levels of oestrogen. But there are many overlaps and you may find that you have several types of hormonal imbalances at work. For example, if you have fibroids, it may be that too much oestrogen in conjunction with too little progesterone could be your problem. PCOS can be associated with either too little or too much oestrogen, depending on how it's affecting you, and generally, because ovulation is a problem, low progesterone is a contributor too.

Reading this section will give you a general idea of how hormonal imbalances work. You will need to read both this chapter, which describes the symptoms associated with hormonal imbalance as well as the contribution made by stress, diet, exercise etc., in conjunction with the section about your particular condition to get a full picture.

1. Too much oestrogen

Many of us are relatively overexposed to the stimulatory effects of oestrogen simply because we have about ten times more periods than our ancestors. Oestrogen excess does not happen just because the ovaries make too much oestrogen. The modern lifestyle (you party animal) also seems to slow down the usual process of getting rid of excess oestrogen through the liver and bowel, and to favour higher circulating levels of available oestrogen. Levels of oestrogen that stay too high seem to be significant risks for diseases. The environmental oestrogens are introduced into the body from outside, mostly through food and water, and can stimulate cells in much the same way as the oestrogens made in the body.

Symptoms
Heavier than usual periods, longer than usual periods, and PMS. Oestrogen excess is linked to endometriosis, fibroids, fibrocystic breast disease, breast and endometrial cancer.

Diagnosis
Excessively high levels of oestrogen are comparative to the levels of other hormones and so excess oestrogen cannot be detected on a single blood test for the oestrogen level. It's usually diagnosed by the symptoms.

Possible causes
Women who eat more fat have significantly higher blood levels of oestrogen. Obesity can cause high oestrogen levels and interfere with ovulation. The ingestion of introduced chemicals, pesticides, hormones, plastics and preservatives in the food chain can also have an oestrogenic effect.

The medical approach
Doctors acknowledge that oestrogen can be 'proliferative', and if they perceive a problem with this, will probably prescribe oestrogen-blocking drugs such as GnRH agonists and Tamoxifen. (For more info on these look under Drugs in The Medical Approach chapter.)

Natural therapies & self care
- Eat less fat and refined carbohydrate.
- Eat more fibre. Natural fibre as part of whole food is recommended, rather than fibre-only breakfast cereals which provide no other wondrous nutrients. See the

20 Good-Eating Hints in the Self Care chapter for more info on fibre.

- Eat more cultured milk products and real yoghurt. Researchers found that eating these foods is associated with lower incidence of breast cancer which they attributed either to the reduced reabsorption of oestrogen or to other immune-enhancing effects of the lactobacillus bacteria.

- Eat more plant oestrogens, like soya products, ground linseeds and sprouted alfalfa. A whole section on these plant oestrogens is in the Natural Therapies chapter.

- Eat up the cabbage family. It helps break down oestrogens in the body. This includes green, purple and white cabbages, broccoli, brussels sprouts and radicchio.

- Look at your protein intake. Higher intakes of protein improve metabolism of oestrogen in the liver. Try to get most of your protein from grains, legumes and low-fat meat and keep it down to 60 grams a day. See the 20 Good-Eating Hints in the Self Care chapter for more info on protein.

- Take vitamin B6. In vitamin B6 deficiency, tissues in the uterus and breast are more susceptible to the stimulating effects of oestrogen, and sadly, B6-deficient women with breast cancer have a poorer survival rate.

- Cut down on alcohol. Moderate alcohol consumption (one glass of beer, one glass of wine or one shot of spirits daily) has been linked to a lower incidence of uterine cancer (particularly in overweight women); but an increased risk of breast cancer. If you have other risk factors for breast cancer it's probably best to cut

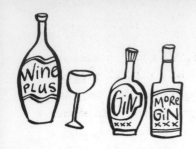

right down on alcohol. Other women, including anyone with an increased risk of heart disease, can safely drink one to two standard glasses every second or third day.

- Moderate exercise helps to reduce the production of oestrogen and increase its clearance from the body.
- Foods which help the liver break down oestrogen include beans, legumes, onions, and garlic.
- Bitter green leafy vegetables and bitter herbs prescribed by a herbalist will help liver function, which may help clear excess oestrogen.
- Reduce pesticide use in your home and garden and campaign for the same in your local area.
- Buy fresh, non-packaged food. (Fatty foods like cheeses, wrapped in cling wrap, can absorb oestrogen-like components from the plastics.)
- Buy foods packaged in glass rather than in plastic or polystyrene.
- Buy organic foods if you can, especially organically grown or range-fed meats.

2. Not enough oestrogen

A relative oestrogen deficiency happens when too much oestrogen is cleared by the body; too little is recycled for use by the body; and/or the fat cells aren't making enough oestrogen from the androgen hormones.

An *actual* oestrogen deficiency happens after menopause, when your ovaries stop making it.

Symptoms

Low bone density, poor fertility, low sex drive, irregular periods, and premature ageing or excessive dryness and brittleness of tissues including vagina, bones and skin.

Possible causes

A body-fat composition of less than 22 per cent can often stop periods and cause oestrogen levels to fall below normal. The cycle can also become erratic, and fertility and bone density are also reduced. (See Being Underweight later in this section.)

Too much fibre lowers oestrogen levels and may increase your chances of developing osteoporosis. Avoid eating lots of wheat-bran only cereals. Fibre taken as part of whole food isn't a problem.

Vitamin A deficiency causes low oestrogen. You can get levels up by eating more betacarotene in orange, yellow and green vegetables or fruits. (Taking vitamin A supplements is not safe during pregnancy.)

Antibiotics reduce substantial numbers of the gut bacteria needed to convert oestrogen into a more active form for use in the body. Yoghurt and cultured milks can eventually improve bowel colonies, but it's better to avoid antibiotics, except in severe infection.

Overexercising reduces the levels of circulating oestrogens, and can cause stopped periods and low bone density.

Smoking alters the metabolism of oestrogen so that more of the inactive oestrogen is produced. If you smoke, you'll be relatively oestrogen deficient, and have an earlier menopause and an increased risk of bone fractures.

The medical approach

If a doctor perceives there is a problem, the Pill or hormone replacement therapy (HRT) will probably be prescribed. The Pill is fully explored under Drugs in The Medical Approach chapter. HRT is covered comprehensively in the sister book in this series, *Menopause*.

Natural therapies & self care

- Follow the obvious path suggested by possible causes listed above, like not overexercising or getting too thin, eating a moderate fibre intake, avoiding cigarettes and antibiotics, and making sure you don't have a vitamin A deficiency.
- Eat food from plants which contain oestrogens. There's a whole section on plant oestrogens in the Natural Therapies chapter.
- Eat foods containing steroidal saponins. Substances called saponins in foods and herbs seem to improve mineral uptake, and can lower blood cholesterol levels. Foods with saponins include soya products, all legumes and potatoes with their skins on.
- You may be prescribed herbs containing high levels of steroidal saponins, including *Chamaelirium luteum*, *Trillium erectum*, *Dioscorea villosa* and *Aletris farinosa*. Some of these seem to have definite oestrogen-like and hormone balancing effects. Herbs are explored in the Natural Therapies chapter.

3. Not enough progesterone

By far the most common problem with progesterone is too little rather than too much. Progesterone is produced by the corpus luteum, the remnant of the egg sac after it has released the egg at ovulation. So the first obvious suspicion is that if you don't have enough progesterone, you probably haven't been up to speed in the egg dispatch department.

Symptoms
Related conditions include PMS, unusual bleeding patterns, lumpy or painful breasts and some types of infertility.

Possible causes
No ovulation. Ovulation fails and no progesterone is produced by the body in the second half of the cycle, the luteal phase. This is a normal, temporary state after child-birth, miscarriage, a pregnancy termination, after stopping the Pill, and while breastfeeding. It is also seen in dysfunctional bleeding patterns, after stress, and around the menopause and the first period.
Luteal phase defects. After ovulation, the remnant egg sac (corpus luteum), is supposed to secrete progesterone during the luteal phase of the cycle. Instead of func-tioning normally, however, the corpus luteum might secrete progesterone for a shorter period or at lower levels. This is known as corpus luteum insufficiency and can be caused by faulty development of the egg and the corpus luteum. Another cause might be failure of hypo-thalamic-pituitary function, when the message from the brain (hypothalamus and pituitary gland) is not adequate for ovarian function to proceed in the usual manner. Ovarian hormone secretion is affected and progesterone

production is the usual casualty. Prolactin seems to increase when progesterone levels are low, and may be implicated in some of the symptoms, such as breast soreness. Infertility, premenstrual syndrome, abnormal menstrual cycle patterns such as dysfunctional uterine bleeding and benign breast disease are believed to be linked to this kind of progesterone problem.

Diagnosis
Progesterone deficiency can be diagnosed in a number of ways. A period symptoms diary (there's one on page 15 that you can photocopy) can be filled out daily for one or more months to ascertain the type, severity and timing of symptoms.

Symptoms related to a progesterone deficiency or lack of availability come on only during the luteal phase of the cycle and include tension, irritability, anxiety or other mood changes.

Basal body temperature (taken by mouth thermometer) can be used to determine the availability of progesterone in the luteal phase. The temperature is taken first thing every morning before any activity at all (including talking or rolling over in bed – you may simply reach languidly for the thermometer). A normal, old-fashioned thermometer gives the most accurate reading. The slight, but detectable rise in the temperature in the luteal phase, which indicates progesterone is present, is reliable about three times in four.

The length of the luteal phase can be measured to find out whether progesterone is produced for long enough. The exact date of ovulation is needed and fewer than 11 days from ovulation to the period means you probably have luteal phase defects. Ovulation can be detected using the basal body temperature, a mid-cycle blood or urine test to check for the mid-cycle surge in luteinising hormone (LH), or an ultrasound scan to view the developing follicle.

Blood levels of progesterone are usually taken between seven and nine days after ovulation. But blood tests to determine progesterone levels can get results which fluctuate widely and can range from normal to very low within a short time-span.

A doctor might suggest an endometrial biopsy to evaluate endometrial development, usually performed during a hysteroscopy (explained under Surgery in The Medical Approach chapter). Luteal phase defects are associated with slow maturing of the endometrium.

The medical approach
Many doctors won't perceive progesterone levels as a problem unless ovulation has stopped, and it causes bleeding or infertility. Doctors will often prescribe progestogen drugs, such as Provera, Primulut N and Micronor for dysfunctional uterine bleeding (DUB) caused by not ovulating and low progesterone. Progesterone vaginal suppositories may be prescribed for women who have had several miscarriages, although this is controversial because some miscarriages are a natural way of dealing with a pregnancy which isn't developing normally. More info on progestogens is under Drugs in The Medical Approach chapter.

Natural therapies & self care

- Stress can be a big factor in low progesterone levels and might need to be attended to to improve symptoms.
- A herbalist may prescribe *Vitex agnus castus*, or other herbs which contain steroidal saponins and which seem to normalise ovulation.
- Treatment for symptoms like mood changes is under the PMS section.

LIFESTYLE FACTORS THAT AFFECT YOUR PERIOD

1. Stress

'Stress' is any event or series of events, physical or emotional, in a person's life that leads to physiological and biochemical changes. These events or feelings, either happy or horrible, can include exams, travelling, moving away from home, relationship problems, getting married, getting unmarried, serious illnesses or extreme physical exercise.

Effects on the period

Stress can interfere with normal hormone levels. This can cause periods to stop temporarily; heavier than usual periods; erratic cycles; and dysfunctional uterine bleeding (DUB). Stress can affect fertility by causing ovulation to stop temporarily, or by disrupting the cycle.

PMS can become worse with stress – some researchers even think that most women have some premenstrual symptoms, but stressed and anxious women develop worse

PMS because they are unusually sensitive to hormone fluctuations and find it harder to cope.

Stress increases the perception of pain and blunts your coping skills. It may cause changes in the hypothalamic-pituitary hormones which regulate the menstrual cycle. Some people get worse period pain when they're stressed.

Period pain in some teenagers has been linked to stress caused by family tension, guilty feelings about sex, or being encouraged to think of periods as unclean and a problem. The good news is that the stressful time usually ends and the periods return to normal.

Symptoms

The body's first reaction to stress is an 'alarm' response. Messages from the hypothalamus stimulate the nervous system which in turn stimulates the adrenal glands to produce adrenalin. This leads to a faster heart rate; increased production of sweat; contraction of the spleen to return blood to the circulation; dilation of the pupils, and of the bronchioles in the lungs; and release of stored sugars. Digestion and the production of urine slows down.

This response is the 'fight or flight mechanism' and was much more in demand when it was regularly necessary to go four rounds with a woolly mammoth. A rapid heart rate and contraction of the spleen means that more blood is available for muscles, a sudden burst of glycogen sugar gives instant energy, you can see better, breathe faster and be more alert.

These days, when we get stressed about relationships, work or money, we can't run away screaming or try to bash up a prehistoric elephant. So the excess adrenalin remains circulating in your system, leaving you edgy, or 'wired'. In times of prolonged stress including chronic illness, pain, or emotional trauma, the 'alarm' response changes into the 'resistance' response. Many organs become distracted from their usual jobs by special functions to deal with stress.

The body comes under enormous physical strain and needs a lot more nutrients than usual but the stress makes you lose your appetite, get indigestion and not assimilate nutrients properly. Potassium excretion increases right at the time you need extra help with the normal function of the heart, other muscles, and the nervous system. The combination of hormone production and fluctuating blood sugar levels creates a sense of irritability and sometimes, anxiety attacks. There's often disturbed sleep and night sweats. (Not to be mistaken for menopause!) Functional hypoglycaemia can be a problem too, brought about by the changes in stress hormones and fluctuations in the blood sugar.

Some stresses are just too extreme or go on too long. This leads to the 'exhaustion' phase of the stress response. Many of the organs go into decline, minerals are excreted in the urine, the immune response weakens, sleep is unrefreshing and often disturbed by weird dreams about octopus wrestling (or that kind of thing) and you feel exhausted and daunted all the time. Other symptoms include being depressed, moody, anxious and unable to remember anything. Utterly repressible.

The medical approach

Few modern doctors are still keen to prescribe some dubious tranquillisers. These drugs are not appropriate for temporary, stress-related changes to your period. Stress management techniques are favoured by most doctors and natural therapists.

Natural therapies

All the following herbs must be prescribed by a herbalist specialising in menstrual problems. You can't go ferreting around with them on your own.

- A group of herbs called the adaptogens helps the body adapt to stress. This group of herbs includes the ginsengs, especially *Eleuthrococcus senticosus*.
- Nervine herbs are also useful when sleep is disrupted, along with B vitamins, and magnesium supplements taken in the mornings. Some herbalists prescribe an extract of the green oat seed (to be taken in a liquid herbal mixture) or *Hypericum perforatum* for depression.
- Herbs which regulate periods after stressful episodes are *Vitex agnus castus* for erratic periods and PMS; *Cimicifuga racemosa* (especially if you're approaching menopause); and *Leonurus cardiaca* and *Verbena officinalis* for period irregularities linked with anxiety and palpitations.

Self care

- Try the dietary guidelines for hypoglycaemia (pages 184–8) which will improve many of your symptoms, and your ability to cope with long-term stress.

- Avoid stimulants such as coffee, alcohol, cigarettes, and wild affairs in the Bahamas.
- Adopt stress management techniques such as yoga, 'long slow distance' exercise, relaxation tapes or meditation. (If you're bored with the idea of meditation, anything that makes you have fun or feel relaxed will do, which is where a wild affair in the Bahamas might come in handy.)
- If your budget doesn't quite stretch to lust in the distant tropics, try herbal teas such as chamomile and lime flowers, which can be mixed together. Lemon balm tea is useful for stomach upsets caused by anxiety, especially when combined with chamomile tea.
- Eat oats or porridge, it's good for the nervous system.
- Rub a little oil of ylang ylang or lavender (diluted in a base oil such as olive oil) on your temples to reduce anxiety. Some people find these oils useful for tension headaches. You can also use a few drops in an atmospheric oil burner floating on water, or in the bath (Whatever you do, don't swallow essential oils.)
- Rescue Remedy, a Bach flower essence available from health food shops and most natural therapists, is useful to relieve anxiety caused by one-off worrying events like exams or public speaking. It can also be used for sleeplessness caused by worry.
- Improve sleep by getting to bed at the same time each night and having a lavender-scented bath and a warm drink like soya or cow's milk with honey.

2. Dieting and fasting

Effects on the period

Dieting to lose weight has its merits — almost everyone does it at some stage or another, but care should be taken not to adopt a diet that is detrimental to good health. Dieting can adversely affect the period, but often the changes are more subtle than those as described below. Seek professional advice when going on a diet that you intend to stay on for longer than a month. Check whether it contains everything you need every day. If you're an adolescent, breastfeeding, pregnant, exercising heavily, have heavy periods or are convalescing, you will need modifications to the regular recommendations for other women.

Beware of diets that also restrict the intake of essential nutrients such as calcium and iron. Many women who are chronic dieters have very low dietary calcium intakes and are finding that their bone density has been adversely affected over the long term. It makes no sense to main tain a suitable body weight or to reduce the risk of heart disease, for example, and then to end up with osteoporosis as a trade-off. Iron is another common deficiency for dieters. Chronically low iron causes anaemia which can be associated with fatigue and dizziness and can cause heavier periods. This can also be caused by diets that result in a deficiency in bioflavonoids and vitamin A.

Be very cautious of extreme dietary restrictions. These usually follow two types of broad recommendations — either fasting, detox diets or restricted eating on one hand, or favouring one type of food, usually at the expense of a well-balanced diet, on the other. These types of diets each have their own areas of concern and need to be looked at separately.

Fasting, cleansing and detox diets

As a general rule, if you're tired, run-down or feeling depleted in any way, then you should go on a regime to build yourself up before attempting to go on any detox or 'elimination' regime. So if you are run-down, especially after the birth of a child, a serious illness, recovering from surgery or having dealt with an episode of severe or prolonged stress and someone tells you to detox or fast, seek advice from a practitioner who will attend to your depleted state first.

Fasting, raw food only or 'elimination' diets are usually advised for some form of cleansing or purification and may be promoted for just about any type of illness by the radical fringe of the 'natural health' movement. Of greatest concern are those diets that aim to purify or 'cleanse' the system so that the period flow is stopped or dramatically reduced. The idea here is that periods are somehow impure. The argument — usually implied — is that if you have difficult periods, or bleed heavily, or even have periods at all, you're in some way 'toxic' and in need of a detoxifying regime. Someone ought to tell them that the Middle Ages is, like, over. Prolonged restricted diets can reduce or stop periods, not because the body is cleansed or purified, but because the weight is too low to ovulate and get a period.

We hasten to add that not all types of cleansing diets are a hopeless waste of time or dangerous. A well-managed detox diet can be very useful for a variety of complaints, but is usually only warranted for short bursts under supervision to attain a therapeutic goal, and definitely not as a long-term regime. These diets might, for example, consist of a high intake of vegetables, fish, yoghurt; a restricted intake of fruit and starchy foods; with complete abstinence from coffee, tea and alcohol. They generally last for about one week and might be recommended, for example, for someone who has developed chronic thrush, as a prelude to a better eating and lifestyle regime. Fasting is pretty much out of vogue these days (apart from for religious reasons) because it has been shown that not eating at all actually slows down the body's ability to detoxify itself.

Finally, not all diets will suit everyone and will usually need to be adapted to suit each individual body's strengths and weaknesses. For example, the ever-popular 'Liver Cleansing Diet', while offering some sensible advice on how to tidy up your diet, can also cause a variety of problems for some. Vegetables and lemon juices in the morning can give some people diarrhoea and an upset stomach. If this is you, it's best to leave the juices alone or include them in the late afternoon before dinner. Many people who go on this diet unsupervised are also not getting enough calcium, and if there are special needs in this regard, the diet must be adjusted accordingly. Yoghurt is a good addition; especially low fat, to keep saturated fat intake to a minimum. It helps with digestion as well as calcium intake.

High fibre and restricted carbohydrate diets

Fibre recommendations for the average woman are around 30 grams daily, but higher levels of say up to 40 grams might be recommended for women with polycystic ovarian syndrome (PCOS – there is a full section on this later on). Diets with a higher level of fibre are not usually recommended, but sometimes they can be mistakenly suggested as a good way to lose weight. Stay away from this option as the trade-off in the reduction of overall health is too costly. Too much fibre in the diet can cause light periods and damage bone density because it reduces the availability of oestrogen.

Another 'new' fad diet is the high protein, low or no carbohydrate diet recommended for weight loss. Used over a protracted length of time, these diets can cause bowel problems because of the lack of fibre. Another unwanted effect is that they tend to be higher in animal fats than a well-rounded diet and with the additional lack of fibre, can result in a rise in cholesterol. This is particularly a problem for women in their forties, but should be a concern for all women. The higher animal fat intake can also cause heavier and more painful periods because of the imbalance in saturated fats and essential fatty acids. (See the section on Bad Fats and Good Fats in the Self Care chapter.)

Self care

- Avoid restricted diets of any kind unless they are for a special, therapeutic reason, such as treating hypoglycaemia. They should always be used under professional supervision.

- Steer clear of food fad theories which don't include food from all food groups, whether they're in magazines, 'natural health' literature or advice from practitioners. Be especially scornful of 'one food'-type diets, like all fruit and vegetable or all cheese or all banana daiquiris.
- Remember that short-term diets to reduce weight are unsuccessful; the weight always comes back. A long-term change in eating habits is needed, with the aim of gradual change.
- Any weight-loss program must include sensible exercise.

3. Being underweight

Being underweight is a very common cause of period disruptions. It's defined as having a body-fat composition of less than 22 per cent. One of the ways to tell if body weight is within the normal range for your height is to calculate your Body Mass Index (BMI).

To calculate your BMI, divide your weight in kilograms by your height in centimetres squared.

For example, if you weigh 52 kilos and your height is 1.7 metres, you divide the weight (52) by the square of your height (1.7 times 1.7 is 2.89). The answer to the calculation is 17.99. Rounded up to the nearest full number, your BMI is 18, and that puts you in the underweight category.

Roughly speaking, on the BMI scale:
- Less than 20 is considered to be underweight.
- 20—25 is normal.
- 26—30 is overweight.
- Over 30 is considered to be obese.

Each of the categories of the BMI spans a number of kilograms. So if your body frame is very large, you should take the reading from the upper level of the scale and vice versa. And don't forget that calculating your BMI means nothing at all until you've gained full height — that is usually around 20 years of age.

Effects on the period

We each need fat to make up about 17 per cent of our total body weight, or we won't be able to have a period at all. We need about 22 per cent body fat to have periods regularly. On average, we stop having periods once our body-fat composition is below 15–20 per cent of our total body weight. Many underweight girls and women stop having periods, including sportswomen, gymnasts, ballet dancers and dieters.

When you're underweight, hormone levels drop, and ovulation stops as well as the period. Bones and other tissues that depend on oestrogens begin to weaken and you may develop osteoporosis quite early in life. In addition, menopausal symptoms could develop, such as hot flushes and vaginal dryness.

Causes

Extreme weight loss can be caused by serious illnesses such as cancer, malabsorption syndromes and severe dysentery. The most common cause, though, is undereating or overexercising without eating enough good food. Young women who suddenly become vegetarian or vegan can sometimes lose too much weight if they don't know how to manage these diets properly. ('I'm a vegetarian — so

I'll just have a packet of Twisties, some gummy bears and a milk shake.') Some people believe that they should be very thin to be attractive, or healthy – both of these ideas are untrue. Sometimes they find it hard to believe that they are 'too thin' instead of needing to lose more weight. We need to understand that we are all meant to be different healthy, gorgeous shapes and sizes. And if you have stopped having periods and then when you put on some healthy weight your periods come back, it means you were too thin for you.

The medical approach, natural therapies & self care
- You'll be encouraged to understand what is a healthy weight range for you, individually and never mind what Cindy Crawford looks like – the woman has different genes entirely. (We pause here for a short plug for Kaz's book about how to feel good about your natural size and shape, *Real Gorgeous: The truth about body and beauty*, published by Allen & Unwin.)
- Read the info on food and diet in the Self Care chapter of this book, and follow the advice. Don't let yourself go hungry.
- Don't go on short-term weight-loss or so-called 'purifying' diets!

4. Being obese
This is nothing to do with 'feeling too fat'. And it is a different category to overweight. 'Obese' is a medical definition that is probably best diagnosed by applying the Body Mass Index (BMI) calculations (see page 51).

Effects on the period

Obesity can cause heavier periods, and alter the menstrual cycle in unpredictable ways. It also gives you an increased risk of breast and endometrial cancer, because more oestrogen is made in the fat cells and those cancers are linked to high oestrogen levels. Usually, obesity will also mean a low level of sex hormone binding globulins in the blood, and this can mean that androgen hormones are freed up to cause symptoms like excess hairiness.

The medical approach

Some doctors prescribe diet pills, but most doctors are coming to realise the dangerous side effects of diet pills including liver damage, drug dependence and wild mood swings. Doctors will usually recommend long-term adjustment of eating habits and a program of exercise. Short-term weight-loss diets are notoriously unsuccessful, and there is evidence that they actually encourage extra weight gain because of changes to the body's metabolism. A nutritionist can help set you up with a long-term eating plan and exercise program. Your doctor can refer you to somebody local.

Natural therapies

Obesity leads to insulin resistance and a natural therapist might suggest you follow a diet like the one described on page 190 in the Natural Therapies section. You are also likely to be given advice on exercise and supplements. Some herbs are helpful, but are not a weight-loss method in themselves and shouldn't be prescribed as such.

Self care

- Don't go on short-term diets.
- Beware of all the 'quick-fix' methods advertised such as so-called 'slimming teas' and 'meal replacements'. There is no magic potion.
- Don't leave a gap of more than 5 hours between meals, preferably less.
- Drink water rather than sugary drinks, tea or coffee.
- Exercise is essential, but seeking professional help at some stage may be a good option. Try starting out with walking for half an hour every second day and slowly increasing the time and the speed of the walk.
- If there is an underlying psychological problem you'd like to tackle, seek professional help from a specialist counsellor.

5. Not exercising
Effects on the period
Not exercising at all isn't much good for anything. Exercise can reduce or fix period pain, improve PMS symptoms and even reduce period flow.

Regular exercise cuts the incidence of other gynaecological problems too, and may lower the risk of endometriosis because it probably slows down oestrogen production. The incidence of endometriosis increases among women who lead bum-sitting lives and among younger women who stop exercising earlier than their peers. Premenstrual sore breasts and cystic disease of the breast are also less likely if you exercise moderately and regularly.

Self care

We pause for a short disclaimer: in case you already have a medical condition, check with your health professional before suddenly hurling yourself about in a frenzy of exercising. Now: the 'moderate exercise' needed to get benefits in the menstrual department might be as little as half an hour a few times a week; period pain and PMS can even improve if you exercise only during the week leading up to the period.

Exercise which increases the heart rate (aerobic exercise) like walking, swimming, cycling, jogging, team sports or aerobics deliver the most all-round benefits, but anything will do.

Specific yoga exercises which improve pelvic blood flow can be a great help with period pain. Yoga often includes relaxation skills, useful to help cope with pain and PMS. These exercises can be taught by a yoga teacher or learned from a book with specific exercises for the pelvic region.

The best de-stressing exercise is a long, slow, distance exercise (called LSD, apparently, if you can believe it). This is when rhythmic and repetitive exercise, usually walking, bike-riding or swimming, is sustained at a moderate pace for between 45 minutes and an hour. This calms the nerves, shuts off the inappropriate adrenal response and improves stamina.

Any weight-bearing exercise, but particularly types which stress the large muscles, has the potential to improve bone mass. The best types are walking, running or playing sport. Swimming and cycling are still important even though they are not classically included in the weight-bearing group.

For maximum benefit, exercise should be daily or every second day for about an hour.

Staying fit and active is important for older women too. Muscle strength and physical fitness increases bone mineral density, improves agility, and cardiovascular health, and reduces your chances of falling and serious injury.

For beginners, quick walking for half to one hour every second day and then every day as stamina improves is an easy way to start.

A good book for extra reading and strategy ideas is *Strong Women Stay Young* by Miriam E. Nelson, published by Lothian.

6. Too much exercise
Effects on the period
Overexercising can cause many problems with the menstrual cycle throughout life. In teenagers it can delay the period and puberty, including growing to normal height. Infertility is also common because ovulation is either erratic or stops. Another big worry is the possibility of irreversible changes to bone density. This can lead to: a failure to reach peak bone mass, reduced bone density, spinal curvature, and stress fractures in the bones.

Women who engage in strenuous physical activity during the period have an increased risk of endometriosis, thought to be related to the increased amount of blood going back up the Fallopian tubes.

If you do prolonged, over-rigorous or endurance exercise, a reversible oestrogen deficiency can develop, which stops ovulation and periods. This could be the body's way of avoiding pregnancy in times of stress and physical endurance.

This stopping of the period by overexercising can be influenced by other factors. Young women who start to overexercise before their first period or before their cycle is properly established are inclined to delay their first period. And if the heavy training starts about the same time as the first period, a history of missed periods is more likely to develop. If you already have irregular menstrual cycles, light periods or missed periods, overexercising will continue the problem. If you're underweight or you lose heaps of weight during training you'll be more likely to get period irregularities. Not getting enough kilojoules or minerals to replace what exercising uses up will increase the chances of period disorders. The further you run, the more likely you are to get problems with your period. Women who run more than 80 kilometres per week are more likely to have no periods. Runners, gymnasts and ballet dancers are more likely to have no periods than swimmers.

The medical approach
If you are 'addicted' to exercise or do too much, you may need to be referred for specialist counselling. If you have prolonged period irregularities or absent periods, consider the Pill if your bone density is also low.

Natural therapies & self care
- Don't overdo it.
- Athletes need to eat a balanced diet and enough of it to maintain enough body fat, still get their period and

protect bone density. This is often in conflict with coaching advice and sometimes a decision must be made between continuing wellbeing and sporting goals. The Self Care chapter has 20 Good-Eating Hints to help.

- During exercise you have an increased need for most minerals, especially calcium, iron, zinc, magnesium and potassium. A deficiency may contribute to the delayed physical development and period problems. Take calcium supplements in the range of 1–1.5 grams a day – the higher range is necessary when periods are erratic or stopped. Info pages on calcium, zinc, iron and magnesium are under Minerals in the Self Care chapter.

- Endurance training will need to be balanced by additional complex carbohydrates to meet the kilojoule requirements.

- Including plant oestrogens in the diet may also be a help. There's a whole section on these plant oestrogens in the Natural Therapies chapter.

PRESCRIBED DRUGS

Effects on the period

Some drugs increase period flow, others reduce it; some influence the regularity of the cycle; and some can even stop periods temporarily. Not all drug influences are negative – some drugs are deliberately prescribed to re-establish period flow and regularity; and to reduce pain or heavy flow.

The common drugs used for 'women's problems' that might influence your menstrual cycle are the Pill, the progestogens, the GnRH agonists, prostaglandins inhibiting drugs and tamoxifen. There is more info on them, including possible side effects, under Drugs in the Medical Approach chapter.

Other classes of drugs that can affect the period are the steroids such as prednisolone, (Solone), hydrocortisone (Hysone), betamethasone (Celestone) and dexamethasone (Decadron); anticoagulants; and the cytotoxic drugs used for cancer.

Self care
Make yourself aware of any effects on your cycle likely to be caused by drugs you have been prescribed. Change drugs if you can. Ask your doctor or natural therapist to help you offset any annoying or avoidable side effects.

NON-PRESCRIPTION DRUGS

Effects on the period
All 'social' and illegal drugs can affect hormones. These effects can translate into more serious problems such as osteoporosis and infertility.

Coffee is linked to infertility. It can increase period pain, especially if you drink it while you have your period. If you have endometriosis, too much alcohol can stop ovulation and cause infertility, and grog increases the risk of developing endometriosis by about 50 per cent. Alcoholism increases the chance of breast cancer and early menopause, and can also increase prolactin production. High prolactin can be related to erratic cycles, heavy or stopped periods.

Cigarette smoking lowers oestrogen levels, and is related to an increased incidence of irregular periods, infertility and earlier menopause.

Cocaine can elevate prolactin levels and cause abnormal menstrual cycles.

Methadone (and possibly other opiates) increases prolactin levels, but doesn't seem to have long-term effects on ovulation.

Self care
Knock it off.

Okay, it's not that easy. But you might be surprised at how much help is available, including support groups of other people who've been through it.

Many counselling and other services are available. You can start with the Drug and Alcohol Foundation in your area or your local hospital or doctor

PMS: The Premenstrual Syndrome

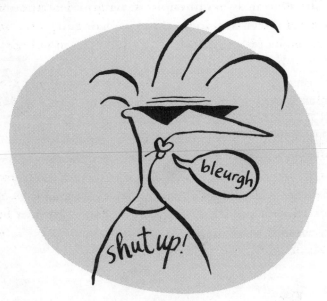

Aarrrgghhhhhhhh!!! Ah yes, the rallying cry of premenstrual women everywhere and here's the rallying cry of the people who have to live with them: 'Get out of the house! Save yourselves!' There are some women who sail through the time before their period being unbelievably jolly and robust, and for the purposes of this chapter we shall ignore them entirely.

Usually in the week or two before their period, premenstrual women can become grumpy, tearful, have a bloated stomach and breasts, get ravenous cravings for Tim Tams, any other sort of food and maybe when that runs out, the furniture, come over all fainty or clumsy or self-hating and generally feel like the world is ending and it's probably not such a bad idea come to think of it. There are many families, housemates and partners who mark red-letter days in their calendar or hang a red scarf from the kitchen light fitting to warn everyone of the vile horrors to be expected.

The good news is that most premenstrual symptoms can be treated — once the right treatment for the individual symptoms is worked out.

PMS (premenstrual syndrome) and PMT (premenstrual tension) are really interchangeable terms, but some people use the term PMT to describe only the emotional symptoms — like tension, irritability and tearfulness. To avoid this confusion, we'll go with PMS to describe both the emotional and physical symptoms known to the vast scary army of the premenstrual.

SYMPTOMS

We mightn't know exactly what causes it, but we know how it makes us feel. A rather ostentatious 150 different symptoms have been recorded in association with PMS. Luckily, no-one gets all of them at once. Most women have their own little collection of regular PMS symptoms, with the occasional extra one. Symptoms might also change after a major biological event, such as childbirth or illness, and you tend to develop different types of symptoms as you approach menopause. Premenstrual headaches, for example, can become more common.

But it is the timing that tells whether you have PMS. There should be no symptoms in the week after the period, but symptoms appearing at any time in the two weeks before a period, and then declining when the period starts.

Some women seeking treatment for PMS, genuinely believing that their mood swings are 'hormonal' find instead they have 'menstrual distress syndrome' or 'menstrual magnification'. Their symptoms are present all month, but get worse before a period. A really useful treatment must tackle the anxiety or depressive state which precedes each period.

The symptoms of functional hypoglycaemia can be easily confused with PMS because of the similarity of the symptoms. If functional hypoglycaemia is the problem, the symptoms will not vary dramatically during the month.

Health practitioners will usually exclude other possibilities as the cause of your symptoms, and see how you respond to treatment for hypoglycaemia.

The most effective way to manage functional hypoglycaemia is changing what and how you eat. In consultation with your health practitioners, follow the dietary guidelines, on pages 184–8 in the Natural Therapies chapter, very strictly for about three weeks and then you can be a bit more relaxed with it, depending on the severity of the problem and how your body responds to the new diet.

Chromium, niacinamide, and magnesium supplements improve functional hypoglycaemia. Some commercially available formulas are specially designed to treat blood sugar problems, and may contain a combination of minerals and vitamins. Follow the instructions on the bottle.

Most common physical symptoms of PMS
- abdominal distension, bloating and discomfort
- breast swelling, pain, discomfort and/or painful, benign breast lumps
- headaches
- abnormal appetite, craving for sweet foods, alcohol and/or fatty foods
- fatigue and weakness
- weight gain of more than 2 kilos
- fluid retention
- premenstrual acne
- joint pains and/or backache
- pelvic discomfort or pain
- increased incidence of upper respiratory tract infections, including sinusitis and recurrent colds
- premenstrual genital herpes outbreaks, recurrent vaginal thrush and/or other infections
- change in bowel habit
- palpitations
- dizziness or fainting
- altered libido

Most common emotional and mental symptoms of PMS
- nervous tension
- mood swings
- irritability
- anxiety

65

- depression
- tearfulness
- confusion
- aggression
- lack of concentration
- forgetfulness
- insomnia

PMS sub-groups

To try and break it down a bit, PMS has been divided into five sub-groups by a research doctor, each based on a different hormonal, biochemical and/or nutritional cause. They are:

- PMS A (A for anxiety) associated with nervousness and irritability;
- PMS C (C for cravings) related to premenstrual sugar cravings and hypoglycaemic symptoms;
- PMS D (D for depression) associated with depression and withdrawal;
- PMS H (H for hyperhydration) where fluid retention is the main symptom; and
- PMS P (P for pain).

Some women with PMS may recognise themselves in more than one of the sub-groups. Treatment for each one is set out below.

Diagnosis

There are no blood tests that can diagnose PMS. The best diagnostic method is to photocopy and fill in the menstrual symptom diary which outlines the classical symptoms: it's in the What is a Normal Period? chapter.

The diary should reveal the timing which suggests PMS — no symptoms after the period; and an increase in symptoms in the two weeks before the period. It may help you find your category of PMS, or rule out PMS.

THE MEDICAL APPROACH

The medical treatment of PMS concentrates on relieving symptoms with diuretics for retained fluid (they can make you wee what seems about a million times so don't take them at night), prostaglandins-inhibiting drugs or anti depressants. The other medical focus is on the manipulation of the hormones with drugs that disrupt ovulation (the Pill, Danazol, GnRH agonists) because if you don't ovulate you don't get PMS, or selectively target one of the abnormal hormones (Bromocriptine). This last drug approach is rare. Many of these drugs have hefty side effects, and should be avoided if possible, as treatment for PMS. Just treating the symptoms is not acceptable for many women and hormonal manipulation can have risks and side effects, so many doctors lean towards the natural therapy approach, and suggest drug therapy only if you don't respond.

NATURAL THERAPIES

Treatments for PMS are based on the five different sub-categories of PMS and are composed of a mixture of supplements and dietary advice, herbal remedies and lifestyle changes.

PMS A (A for anxiety)

This type of PMS is thought to be related to a relative oestrogen/progesterone imbalance, with a relative excess of oestrogen and a relative deficiency of progesterone, possibly related to poor liver clearance of oestrogens, abnormal progesterone production or faulty progesterone receptors.

Symptoms
- nervous tension
- irritability
- mood swings
- anxiety

Treatment
- You may be prescribed a herbal extract of *Vitex agnus castus* berries starting on the first day of the cycle and continuing for between three and six months.
- Vitamin B6: 100–200 milligrams, or vitamin B complex containing 50 milligrams of vitamin B6 for ten to 14 days before the period.
- Magnesium: 200–800 milligrams daily of elemental magnesium in the form of magnesium phosphate, aspartate, orotate or chelate.
- Nevines such as *Valeriana officinalis* (valerian), *Scutellaria laterifolia* (skullcap), *Matricaria recutita* (chamomile) for anxiety.
- *Withania somnifera* for anxiety with exhaustion.
- *Anemone pulsatilla* tincture is especially useful for tension headache with nervousness, especially when combined with *Passiflora incarnata* (passionflower).

- *Betonica officinalis* (wood betony) is used for headache and extreme anxiety, especially in combination with *Scutellaria laterifolia* (skullcap).
- *Bupleurum falcatum*, *Paeonia lactiflora* and *Angelica sinensis* is a common combination used in Chinese medicine for irregular periods with premenstrual anxiety and irritability.
- Plant oestrogens in foods and herbs (more info on plant oestrogens is in the Natural Therapies chapter).
- Herbal and dietary bitters to aid liver clearance of oestrogens.
- Restriction of dairy products and sugar.
- 'Natural' progesterone creams, derived from plants such as *Dioscorea villosa* (wild yam) and soy, are sometimes advocated for the treatment of PMS, but research on its long-term effect is lacking.

PMS C (C for cravings)

PMS C rarely exists as a form of PMS in isolation and often comes with PMS A.

It's linked to functional hypoglycaemia which may be caused by a magnesium deficiency, a sugar-induced sensitivity to insulin, or an imbalance in prostaglandins.

Symptoms
- headache
- increased appetite
- fatigue
- craving for sweets
- palpitations
- dizziness or fainting

Treatment

Blood sugar

- Magnesium: 200-800 milligrams daily of elemental magnesium in the form of magnesium phosphate, aspartate, orotate or chelate.
- Small meals often.
- Restricted sugar and salt intake.
- Dietary and herbal bitters to regulate blood sugar metabolism.

Balancing prostaglandins

- Essential fatty acid supplements, such as evening primrose oil or star flower oil. Doses of 3 grams of evening primrose oil containing 216 milligrams of linoleic acid and 27 milligrams of gamma linoleic acid (GLA) or the equivalent taken daily from mid-cycle until the period may be useful in regulating prostaglandins. You'll need vitamin B6 and zinc to make it work. Diet can also be altered to take in more essential fatty acids. (See Bad Fats and Good Fats in the 20 Good-Eating Hints section of the Self Care chapter.)
- Vitamin E: between 100 and 600 International Units (IU) daily can also help balance prostaglandins.

PMS D (for depression)

This form of PMS is accompanied by depression and withdrawal and is thought to be related to relative oestrogen deficiency. The causes might include lower oestrogen production around the menopause; a depleted oestrogen pool caused by being too thin or eating too much fibre; blocked oestrogen receptors caused by high lead levels; or a progesterone level which is relatively too high.

Symptoms
- depression
- crying
- insomnia
- forgetfulness
- confusion

Treatment
- Magnesium: 200–800 milligrams daily of elemental magnesium in the form of magnesium phosphate, aspartate, orotate or chelate, to decrease lead absorption and retention.
- Eat plant oestrogens (see the plant oestrogen section of the Natural Therapies chapter).
- The 'oestrogenic herbs' which contain steroidal saponins such as *Chamaelirium luteum* (helionias), *Aletris farinosa* (true unicorn root), *Dioscorea villosa* (wild yam), as well as *Angelica sinensis* (Dang Gui) and *Paeonia lactiflora* (white peony).
- *Cimicifuga racemosa*, especially if you get premenstrual headaches.
- *Hypericum perforatum* and *Withania somnifera* for symptomatic treatment of depression.

PMS H (H for hyperhydration)
PMS H is related to fluid retention thought to be brought about by an increase in the adrenal hormone, aldosterone, which is responsible for salt and water retention. This

may be a response to lower progesterone secretion, too much oestrogen, magnesium deficiency, other hormone irregularities, or stress. Prolactin may be implicated when breast soreness is a big symptom.

Symptoms
- breast tenderness
- weight gain
- bloating
- swelling in lower body and eyelids

Treatment
- All treatments for PMS A and those for prostaglandins in PMS C, especially vitamin E: 100–600 IU daily, if breast tenderness is a problem.
- *Taraxacum officinale* leaf (dandelion leaf) as a tea is a mild diuretic and reduces fluid retention. Herbal diuretic tablets are also available.

PMS P (for pain)
In this category of PMS, the major problem is an increased sensitivity to pain which is believed to be caused by prostaglandins imbalance.

Causes are thought to be elevated oestrogen levels, or eating too much animal fat.

Symptoms
- aches and pains
- period pain
- reduced pain threshold

Treatment

- Magnesium reduces sensitivity to pain in doses of 200–800 milligrams daily.
- Essential fatty acids such as evening primrose oil, 3 grams a day, with vitamin B6 and zinc, in doses prescribed by a practitioner. Diet can also be altered to take in more essential fatty acids. (See Bad Fats and Goods Fats, number 8 of 20 Good-Eating Hints in the Self Care chapter.)
- The herb *Tanacetum parthenium* (feverfew) is a prostaglandins-inhibitor and may help with period pain and migraine headaches if taken long term.

SELF CARE

Diet

All types of PMS seem to improve with dietary changes:

- Increase the intake of complex carbohydrates (there's more info on this in the 20 Good-Eating Hints in the Self Care chapter).
- Eat more often — a 'grazing' or hypoglycaemic diet (see the hypoglycaemic diet in the Natural Therapies chapter). Little meals more often is the go. The positive effects may be related to stabilisation of blood sugars as well as to indirect influences on progesterone.
- When fluid retention, bloating and weight gain are problems, cut down on salt — most processed foods, including cheese, are high in salt. Also eat vegetables, grapefruit juice and bananas for potassium.
- If you have breast soreness, muscle or joint pains or period pain you'll probably respond well to reducing

animal fats, processed vegetable oils, coconut, and increasing essential fatty acids and vitamin E. (Essential fatty acids are explained under Bad Fats and Good Fats, number 8 of the 20 Good-Eating Hints in the Self Care chapter.)

- Coffee, alcohol, and chocolate aggravate feelings of depression, irritability and anxiety, as well as worsening many breast symptoms. Leave them alone during the premenstrual phase.
- Many of the symptoms of PMS have been attributed to magnesium deficiency (there's a magnesium info page in the Minerals section of the Self Care chapter). If that sounds like you, eat more magnesium-containing foods and restrict dairy products.
- PMS related to high oestrogen levels relative to other hormones means you need to eat more plant oestrogens. Plant oestrogens also improve symptoms of rapid decline of oestrogens just before the period such as headaches, migraines and depression. (There's a whole section on plant oestrogens in the Natural Therapies chapter.)

Exercise and stress management

Women with PMS who use long slow distance exercise or yoga seem better at handling their physical PMS symptoms. There are suggestions on managing stress in The Usual Suspects section.

Period Pain

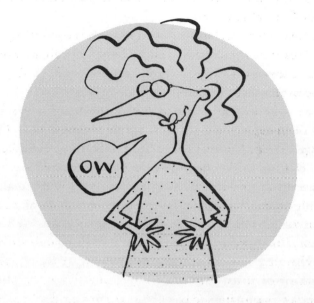

There are legions of washed-out looking women clutching hot-water bottles to their stomachs, dragging around the joint in dressing-gowns and making sure they never run out of painkillers — the ones with 'cramps', or period pain. 'It's that time of the month', they mutter, and everyone nods sympathetically, without even suggesting that a filthy old dressing-gown is not a good look at 4 p.m. Is this something we have to put up with? (The pain, not the dressing-gown.)

Nope. The bottom line here is that pain is, well, a pain. Pain makes people tired and crabby and more likely to go see their health practitioner than any other symptom — maybe it's caused by a disease, maybe by a disorder, maybe by just a slight hormone imbalance that's easy to fix.

Lots of people, some of them doctors and natural therapists, think that a bit of period pain is normal. Patients get used to hearing stuff like, 'Grin and bear it', that hoary old chestnut 'It will be better once you have a baby', and even 'It's just part of being a woman'. Bollocks. It's not something you should put up with, or expect as part of your womanly life. (You're a woman now, and you will have period pain and an automatic instinct for the correct hat for every occasion? Not very scientific.)

The thing is, a bit of period pain is usual, but just because it's common, doesn't mean that it's normal or nothing to worry about. The most important thing about persistent period pain is to find out what's causing it. If your treatments for the pain aren't working, get investigative — it could be a warning from your body about something serious.

The two questions to ask about period pain are: 'Does it bother you enough to want/need to do something about it?' If not, you are excused. Go and sit in the corner and try on some hats until the end of this section. If your period pain is enough to make you do something about it, here's another question: 'Are you happy with the treatments you are using?' If not, read on. It may be well worth your while: after all, on average you have 12 or 13 periods a year, and if you get pain for two or three days, that adds up to a month of pain each year: yikes.

Doctors often call period pain dysmenorrhoea. It sounds rather disgusting, but is basically just ancient Greek for painful periods — *dys* meaning difficulty with, and *menorrhoea* meaning to do with menstruation. It's pronounced Dis-men-oh-rear. Dysmenorrhoea is a symptom, not a disease — so the first aspect of any successful treatment is to find out why you're getting pain.

Period pain falls into two major categories:

· The uterine muscle is behaving abnormally and causing cramps, but is otherwise healthy. This is called naughty uterus. No, it's actually called primary dysmenorrhoea. (Primary dysmenorrhoea is sometimes also called functional dysmenorrhoea. Are they just deliberately trying to confuse us or just SHOWING OFF?)

· A disease of an organ or organs which has pain as one of its symptoms.

This is called secondary dysmenorrhoea. Common causes of secondary dysmenorrhoea include endometriosis and pelvic inflammatory disease (PID).

But sometimes primary dysmenorrhoea can cause really bad pain and secondary dysmenorrhoea is not so bad — that is, really bad pain doesn't automatically mean you have a disease — in fact in some cases disease doesn't cause pain. PID is often called a 'silent' disease because in many cases you don't even know you've got it until you're being tested for infertility.

Before treating your period pain, make sure you get a diagnosis of primary or secondary dysmenorrhoea from your health practitioner.

CAUSES OF 'ORDINARY' PERIOD PAIN

By this, we mean primary dysmenorrhoea, the period pain which is caused by a naughty uterus, not by an underlying 'nasty', like a disease.

A problem with uterine tone

First, a word about where 'cramps' come from. When you have a period, the uterus helps to get the blood out through the cervix and down the vagina by having small contractions.

These muscle contractions continue all the time, even when the uterus is apparently at rest. You just can't feel it. During a period, or childbirth, the uterine activity is amplified many times, but if the period contractions are normal, the pain is not a problem.

The 'resting phase' or 'resting tone' between contractions is important. Normally, the blood flowing through the uterine muscle carries oxygen and other nutrients. When the muscle doesn't rest, the lack of oxygen supply leads to muscle spasm: in other words, cramps. Some women compare this kind of period pain to labour pains. Sometimes the cramping can get so bad it causes severe pain before the period. This usually gets better once the period starts.

Many women also develop diarrhoea, needing to wee all the time, or vomiting – all this is because of the reflex spasm in nearby organs.

The opposite problem can be caused by poor muscle tone in the uterus, accompanied by heavy bleeding or 'flooding' during the period. There may be a sense of heaviness or pelvic congestion, often described as dull, dragging heaviness. Lack of tone can be caused by many pregnancies, recent childbirth and conditions which prevent adequate contraction of the uterus, for example, fibroids, polyps and adenomyosis.

A prostaglandins imbalance

The cause of cramping is usually an imbalance in the prostaglandins levels.

Oh, don't get us started on prostaglandins, they are hideously complicated critters. Suffice to say that prostaglandins are hormone-like substances which are found in most body tissues. Lots of different prostaglandins control several bodily functions by working together as an integrated team. When the prostaglandins are all in balance, the period runs smoothly. But if there are too many of the kind of prostaglandins which increase muscle spasm, then you'll get period cramps.

SYMPTOMS

You name it. Period pain can vary dramatically from person to person, and even from period to period. Some have severe pain that feels sharp, or maybe dull. Others have pain that comes in fits and starts. The most common description of period pain is a continual, dull, 'background' ache or sense of heaviness (someone came over all Greek and called it congestive dysmenorrhoea), also accompanied by episodes of cramping pain (spasmodic dysmenorrhoea).

The pain is usually central and under the navel.

79

Sometimes a heavy aching pain extends to the groin, the back, and down the thighs. Most often, the pain that starts before you see the first blood of the period is congestive and aching. Sometimes this sort of pain is accompanied by a heavy dull sense of dragging in the vagina or a sense of fullness in the bowel. This is the feeling often described as though 'everything will fall out'. (You'll be relieved to know it never does.)

Most often, though, the pain starts with the first blood of the period and intensifies as the flow becomes heavier, or when clots are in the period blood. Usually the spasmodic, crampy-type pain is the shortest part of the pain but it feels the worst.

All that contracting can annoy the neighbours — and the bowel is just next door to the uterus. The bowel tends to be affected by hormone changes too. Many women become constipated before their period and this can exacerbate the sense of fullness and heaviness felt with congestive period pain. Irritable bowel syndrome aggravates period pain and is aggravated by it. The bowel and uterus share a similar nerve supply and when either organ is in spasm, the other will spasm in sympathy. Aaawww.

DIAGNOSIS

Diagnosing ordinary period pain is about exclusion — ruling out other complaints as the origin of the pain. To do this, a health practitioner needs to consider the individual features of your medical, menstrual and obstetric history; your age; and your level and manner of sexual activity. For example, if you've had sex without a condom you have a higher risk of pelvic inflammatory disease, and older women are more likely to have adenomyosis than younger women.

The history of the pain gives other important hints. Relevant clues include: where it is; how long it lasts; which other symptoms accompany the pain; whether it radiates; what treatments have already failed; and whether the pain happens mostly before, during or after bleeding. If you keep a diary which keeps track of these symptoms you will help the diagnosis.

Pelvic examinations

A doctor may suggest an internal examination of the pelvic organs. This usually involves looking at the cervix to see whether it looks normal and healthy, and examining the pelvic organs by inserting a gloved hand into the vagina to feel the size, state and position of the organs. The doctor will be looking for secondary causes of period pain such as an enlarged ovary or uterus, which suggests a problem. Pelvic exams and the reasons they are performed are described in the Screening section of the Medical Approach chapter.

Laparoscopy

Sometimes surgery is needed to make a diagnosis — the operation is usually a laparoscopy, where the surgeon makes two or more small incisions and inserts the laparoscope, a thin pencil-like instrument, to have a look around. It is often recommended if the history is suggestive of secondary causes of pain, or if the pain fails to respond to the medication used for straightforward period pain.

WHEN TO SEE THE DOCTOR

- Your period pain changes in some way or you get period pain for the first time.
- The pain is interfering with your lifestyle.
- Pain is on one side and/or radiating (spreading to the thigh or another area).
- You have pain at the time of your period that is not like your usual period pain, and there's a possibility you might be pregnant.
- Your usual ways of controlling the pain don't seem to work any more.
- New symptoms accompany the pain, for example, vomiting, diarrhoea, or feeling faint.
- The pain gets worse towards the end of the period.
- Pain is aggravated by pressure, bowel motions or sex.
- A fever or discharge accompanies the pain.

Another possible cause of pain

Endometriosis and adenomyosis

Severe period pain could be caused by endometriosis. Endometriosis is a very complex condition and requires specialised care. If you are diagnosed with it or want more information, we humbly suggest you get the book in this series called *Endometriosis* to explain everything. The following symptoms are common if you have endo, so if you do, make doubly sure you get off to the doctor.

These endo symptoms are arranged in order of the most suggestive first:

- really bad period pain
- difficulty getting pregnant
- pain during sex, particularly during penetration
- pain that gets worse towards the end of the period
- pain before the period or at ovulation time
- pelvic pain on one side
- a mother or sister with endo

THE MEDICAL APPROACH TO PAINFUL PERIODS

Prostaglandins-inhibiting drugs like Ponstan are the most likely first suggestion for ordinary period pain, but also common are the Pill and some painkillers. Sometimes, if the pain is severe and fails to respond to the usual treatments, very strong hormone drugs like Duphaston are used.

When period pain is really bad and all other treatments have been unsuccessful, the uterosacral nerve is sometimes cut to destroy the perception of pain in the uterus. This is a drastic last step and is rarely used. If it is recommended to you, we hesitate to say run for the hills, but at the very least get a second opinion.

NATURAL THERAPIES

Everyone experiences period pain differently and has their own combination of symptoms. Herbal formulas which are individually prescribed should try to deal with as many of these symptoms as possible. Over-the-counter herbal remedies for period pain can't have exactly the right combination of herbs for everyone.

It can be quite complicated to design a remedy for period pain. You'll need a specialist herbalist to prescribe your individual formula. You're likely to be prescribed a 'cocktail' of the following herbs, tailored to your individual diagnosis.

The uterine tonics including *Aletris farinosa*, *Caulophyllum thalictroides*, *Angelica sinensis* and *Rubus idaeus*.

The anti-spasmodic herbs including *Viburnum opulus* and *V. prunifolium*, *Caulophyllum thalictroides*, *Dioscorea villosa* and *Paeonia lactiflora*. *Paeonia lactiflora* is usually combined with *Glycyrrhiza glabra* (liquorice) to obtain the best effect. *Caulophyllum thalictroides* is used when the spasm seems to be localised in the cervix, resulting in acute crampy pain with very little flow. Once the flow gets going there should be pain relief.

Emmenagogue, or **expulsive herbs**. This category of herbs especially should only be used by a properly trained herbalist: as Aunty Myrtle always said, never let an amateur near your uterus, dear.

Warming herbs: especially two specific for the pelvic region: *Zingiber officinale* (ginger) and *Cinnamomum zeylanicum* (cinnamon). Both can be added to a herbal mix in the form of a tincture, or taken as a tea, either alone, with other therapeutic herbs or in an ordinary cuppa.

Nervine (relaxing) herbs are useful to help the action of the anti-spasmodic and pain-killing herbs, and also if anxiety or tension accompany the pain. Some nervine herbs are also anti-spasmodics, the best being *Valeriana officinalis, Paeonia lactiflora, Piscidia erythrina, Corydalis ambigua, Verbena officinalis* and *Matricaria recutita* (chamomile).

Anodyne, or pain-reducing herbs. *Corydalis ambigua* from the Chinese *Materia Medica* is the most potent of these, and can be used for pain anywhere in the body. It also reduces heavy period flow. Other important anodynes for period pain are *Piscidia erythrina, Lactuca virosa* and *Anemone pulsatilla*.

Prostaglandins-inhibiting herbs include *Zingiber officinale* (ginger), *Tanacetum parthenium* (feverfew) and *Curcuma longa*. There are probably others, but there is little research in this area.

Herbs which regulate the hormone levels. The most valuable of the herbal hormone regulators is *Vitex agnus castus*, which is very useful for congestive period pain, especially if PMS is also a problem. Vitex is a very difficult herb to prescribe successfully and should be prescribed by a specialist practitioner. Other herbs include *Paeonia lactiflora* and *P. suffruticosa* and *Cimicifuga racemosa* which are anti-spasmodics and may

85 OW

also competitively inhibit the activity of oestrogen; and *Verbena officinalis* which is a sedative and has been traditionally used for hormonal period disorders.

Congestive period pain, the heavy, dull, dragging type of pain experienced by many women before their period, is often improved by taking **liver herbs** or **bitters** such as *Berberis vulgaris* which is also an emmenagogue. Other liver herbs include *Taraxacum officinale* (dandelion), *Silybum marianum* (St Mary's thistle).

For spasmodic or congestive period pain accompanied by constipation and irritable bowel syndrome, the **'aperient' (laxative) herbs** such as *Cassia senna* (senna pods), *Rhamnus purshiana* (cascara) and *Aloe barbadensis* (aloe) can be used. However, these will often aggravate spasm in the uterus if taken during the period. Beware of laxatives bought from the chemist with these elements, as the effects can be rather, ahem, violent.

By far the best method to treat constipation is to increase the level of fibre and fluids in the diet. (There are sensible high-fibre diet suggestions in the Self Care chapter.) Irritable bowel syndrome often becomes worse around the period and can aggravate period pain — sometimes it is even mistaken for period pain.

Acupuncture

Acupuncture can help some period pain. It involves the insertion of needles into the skin which sounds scary, but if you breathe in really quickly as each needle goes in you don't feel a thing. Obviously what you'll need is an experienced acupuncturist, not some mad pal with an old school compass – the placing of the needles is very precise. The treatments are usually given twice a week.

Chiropractic and osteopathy

Some chiropractors and osteopaths believe that period pain can be aggravated by pressure on the spinal nerves that supply the uterus. They treat this problem by manipulating the lower back. Any likely positive response should be obvious within one or two treatments.

SELF CARE

- Cut down on animal fats (especially meat, egg yolk and prawns/shrimps) and increase essential fatty acids in foods. The oil of evening primrose and especially fish oils can improve period pain. Usually a dose of 3 grams a day of either in capsule form is necessary to achieve good results. For the first few months, taking the supplements daily is a good idea. This can be expensive, but the dose can be reduced once pain control is achieved. Try fish oils first. Essential fatty acids are explained under Bad Fats and Good Fats, number 8 of the 20 Good-Eating Hints in the Self Care chapter.
- Calcium and magnesium supplements will sometimes relieve period cramps. Follow the recommended dose on the label. Usually, a combination of calcium and magnesium is best. (An info page on both is in the Minerals section of the Self Care chapter.)
- Relax: it helps you cope with pain. Guided imagery and meditation can be useful as well, if you're into that sort of thing. Guided imagery is when you imagine

yourself to be free of pain – if that works, try imagining you've won the lottery.

- Make ginger tea: grate 2–4 centimetres of fresh root ginger, place in a stainless steel saucepan with one to two cups of water, cover and bring slowly to the boil. Keep covered and simmer for about ten minutes. Strain, add honey to taste and sip while still hot. If possible, also have a warm bath. Other herbs can be taken at the same time. Ginger also eases nausea and is useful for period pain accompanied by nausea and vomiting. Commercial tablets such as Travel Calm (Blackmores), are quite useful for mild period pain.

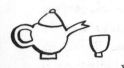

- A therapeutic massage just before or during the period can help. Some specific massage techniques like shiatsu, acupressure, and foot reflexology can be used to relieve pain, pelvic congestion and symptoms of hormone imbalance.
- Try aromatherapy. Clary sage, lavender, and chamomile oil are all useful for period pain because of their anti-spasmodic and relaxing properties.

They can be used regularly in the bath, as a component of massage oil or as a warm compress, but should not be swallowed. These oils are not applied to the skin 'neat', and should be diluted with a base oil such as olive oil, or water.

- To make massage oil, add between 1 and 3 millilitres, or 20 and 60 drops of each essential oil to 100 millilitres of a base oil (olive, almond or apricot kernel oil are good). Massage into the lower abdomen and back when pain is a problem. It may be useful to have a hot bath first, then use the massage oil. You may also find it useful to have the massage done by a large muscly fireman called Sven, who then slowly ... I beg your pardon.

- You can make a hot compress by adding about 5 drops of each essential oil to a bowl of very hot water, soaking a cloth and then applying it to the painful area of the stomach after wringing out the excess water. The cloth can be repeatedly dipped in the water each time it cools. Alternatively, a hot-water bottle can be placed over the compress to keep it warm.

- An aromatherapy bath is easy. Usually only about 5–10 drops are needed in a full bath tub. Valerian oil can be very useful if the period pain prevents sleep, or when it is useful to 'sleep the pain off'. It can make some people quite drowsy, so don't expect to be the life of the party afterwards. (Although we do know of a determined girly who used to take her hot-water bottle with her to the nightclubs and fill it up at the urn.)

- Heat of any sort will help to relieve muscle spasm. A hot-water bottle or a hot bath is cheap and easy. It is also possible to buy small hot packs that can be worn close to the skin – some manu- facturers even sell them with specially made undies with a little pouch to hold the pack in place. ('Warmease' is the name of one product, but try a chemist before the sexy lingerie department.)

- Try a warm ginger pack on the lower abdomen. (It's kind of messy.) Place grated root ginger between several layers of cloth and place a hot-water bottle over the top. A little oil on the skin first will prevent burns from the ginger juice. Remove the pack if the skin starts to burn or sting.

- While warmth is helpful, getting cold can increase pain. Swimming in cold water can be a problem. The swimming itself can relieve pain, so go for a heated pool.
- If your period pain gets worse with exposure to cold, or better with heat, avoid iced drinks, ice cream or food straight from the fridge. Raw foods, like salads, can also be a problem, and raw vegies can bring on irritable bowel syndrome because the stomach has to work harder to digest them. Try warm food at room temperature or hotter; and add warming spices to food, like ginger, cardamom, coriander, turmeric and cinnamon.
- Having sex or an orgasm can sometimes help to reduce period pain by reducing muscle spasm and pelvic congestion. Hotsy totsy!
- There is an ointment you can buy at pharmacies which is made of wild yam cream (not to be confused with natural progesterone) and other herbal extracts. The creams may work because they contain spasmolytic herbs, but there's no reason to rub it in rather than the easier and cheaper method of swallowing a herbal mixture or tablet. Last time we looked, the ointment price was about $45 for two months, and you're supposed to rub it into different parts of your body two to three times a day!

Heavy Periods

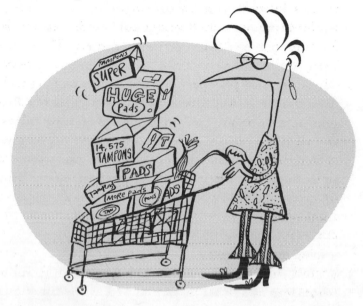

Heavy periods can drive some of us mad: carrying around industrial-strength tampons by the carton load, rushing to the loo every hour or so to check whether there's a 'leak', and knowing, deep in the heart, that popping on a pair of white trousers is about as likely as having Elvis pop in for afternoon tea.

CAUSES OF HEAVY PERIODS

Fibroids are one of the most common causes of heavy periods. But they're not the only cause. Don't let anybody

91

treat your abnormal period bleeding without knowing its cause. An accurate diagnosis is vital. To diagnose fibroids, you'll need to have an ultrasound — and if the bleeding is not caused by fibroids, you may need a whole lot of other tests. Sometimes a diagnosis can be made using only the history of your period patterns, and routine examinations; sometimes you'll need simple surgery, such as laparoscopy or hysteroscopy. (These procedures are explained later in the Medical Approach chapter.) The diagnostic techniques used by natural therapists such as iris, tongue or pulse diagnosis, are much less invasive (and therefore much more fun), but they're often not good enough for what we're dealing with here. They should never be used as an alternative to the appropriate medical examinations.

Functional menorrhagia

The word *menorrhagia* is used by doctors to describe heavy periods as a usual pattern as well as any functional disorder which causes heavy periods. So functional menorrhagia means abnormally heavy periods within a usual cycle length. No disease or problem is revealed from tests on the uterus or blood. The usual medical treatment is going on the Pill, while herbal treatments will need to be individually prescribed.

Endometriosis

This is caused by the endometrium (normal cells lining the uterus) growing elsewhere — on the ovaries, tubes, pelvic ligaments, bowel or bladder. These cells still bleed during periods, often causing cysts, and heavy periods and bad period pain are common. A sister book to this one, called *Endometriosis*, covers the whole shebang.

Adenomyosis

Adenomyosis is like endometriosis but the displaced cells grow in the uterine wall. Their monthly bleeding into the muscle layer causes pain and sometimes heavy periods.

Pelvic inflammatory disease (PID)

PID is caused by infection, which may or may not be sexually transmitted. The symptoms can include abnormal bleeding and heavy periods in about 30 per cent of cases, but more typically cause fever, malaise and pelvic pain. It can also show no apparent symptoms and cause infertility. A bloody or yukky discharge is common if the PID is caused by gonorrhoea, a sexually transmitted disease. PID can be cured with drugs but some damage to Fallopian tubes may be irreversible.

Contraceptives

The IUD or 'loop' can cause heavier and more painful periods. Some women experience bleeding between periods, especially in the first three months after IUD insertion. Severe pain and/or bleeding may indicate that the IUD has dislodged or an infection has developed and requires immediate assessment. Tubal ligation ('having your tubes tied') has been linked to heavy periods. This may be caused because the Pill is stopped after the operation.

Non-gynaecological causes

Disturbance in hormone levels, blood clotting or deficiencies of certain nutrients may result in heavier periods. The more common causes are related to the following systems:

The blood

Disorders of blood production or blood clotting can be related to heavy periods. Causes include anaemia, lack of nutrients (especially iron), blood clotting abnormalities and rare blood disorders.

The endocrine system

Heavy bleeding can be caused by imbalances of the adrenal hormones, from a disorder of the thyroid gland or hypo-thalamic-pituitary unit or as a side effect of drugs on those parts of the body. Most disorders can be controlled by drugs.

The liver

The liver metabolises hormones and has a role in blood clotting. Poor liver function can lead to heavy periods. Improving liver function is a priority for natural therapists.

Pregnancy

Pregnancy-related conditions are the most common causes of abnormal bleeding among women between 20 and 40.

Miscarriage

A late and/or painful, heavy period may be an early miscarriage or a case of the foetus failing to develop normally. Bleeding later in an established pregnancy, and before the fourteenth week, might also be a miscarriage. Sadly, about one in five pregnancies ends in a miscarriage.

FIBROIDS

What are they?

Fibroids are fibrous, non-cancerous growths on the uterus (don't panic if a doctor talks about fibroid tumours, uterine leiomyomas or uterine myomata: it's just the same thing with scarier names). They affect up to a quarter of women over the age of 35. A fibroid is made of dense muscular fibres arranged in circular layers and surrounded by a layer of compressed smooth muscle cells.

Fibroids vary greatly in size, number, and position. Some grow really big and cause pressure symptoms; others stay small and don't cause any problems. It's rare, but very occasionally fibroids can become cancerous.

There are different types of fibroids. They are usually self-contained, fibrous tumours, benign, and roughly spherical. But some are 'pedunculated', attached to the uterine cavity or the outside of the uterus by a stem or 'pedicle'. In rare cases these can twist on the pedicle (called torsion). This can cause extreme pain. Immediate surgery may be needed. Fibroids can either grow inside the uterus, just under the inner lining (the endometrium); in the muscle wall of the uterus; or on the outside of the uterus.

Fibroids may cause few symptoms; occasionally quite large ones are discovered because of a routine examination or ultrasound scan for another reason. Fibroids that don't interfere with fertility or cause unwanted symptoms should be left to their own devices and be regularly monitored.

Some measures to reduce too much oestrogen in relation to progesterone can hold their growth steady and reduce the risk of growing more of them.

The ones that need closest monitoring are fibroids which are large, growing on a pedicle or protruding down through the cervix. Yukko. Fibroids that are growing quickly are at an increased risk of developing into an aggressive type of cancer, and often doctors suggest that they be surgically removed to be on the safe side.

Fibroids are much more likely to cause problems with bleeding if they distort the lining of the uterus by growing into the uterine cavity. An ultrasound will pick this up.

Symptoms

The most common symptom of fibroids is heavy periods. Larger fibroids can cause a feeling like you need to wee a lot, pressure, and a feeling of heaviness, dragging and congestion in the lower abdomen. In rare cases, pressure on the ureter (the tube between the kidney and the bladder) may force a back-flow of urine causing structural abnormalities of the kidney and ureter, and abnormal kidney function. Very large fibroids may cause a bulging stomach. Sometimes fibroids will cause a miscarriage or infertility and in rare cases, they may cause early labour.

What makes them grow
Nobody really knows exactly, but we do know that fibroid growth is dependent on oestrogen: they rarely develop before the first period and almost always shrink after menopause. You are at greater risk of fibroids if you have another condition of oestrogen overactivity, such as endometrial hyperplasia or endometriosis. Lowering 'excess' oestrogen is important for a successful treatment.

Fibroids have also been found to contain larger amounts of the chemical DDT than other uterine tissue. The significance of this is not clear, but DDT has oestrogen-like effects and may in some way initiate the tissue changes.

Related factors
Pregnancy seems to reduce the risk of fibroids developing and each pregnancy further reduces the risk.

It's possible that coffee increases the risk of developing uterine fibroids.

Studies which have investigated the Pill and fibroids have been inconclusive: some studies show a reduced incidence; one study shows a slightly increased rate (not statistically significant); and two others found no change. That's a fat lot of good, then.

Diagnosis
A fibroid could be suspected if you also have these signs and symptoms:

 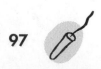

- Heavy periods.
- A sense of congestion in the lower abdomen before and during a period.
- An enlarged uterus discovered by a doctor during a pelvic examination.
- A lower abdominal mass felt by you or your doctor.

An ultrasound scan is used to diagnose uterine fibroids. (Ultrasounds are explained under Screening in The Medical Approach chapter.) They will show up as a shape in or on the uterus. Usually there's a really good view and they can tell you the exact size and position. Ultrasounds are a good way to monitor the growth rate of fibroids.

Some doctors will also want to perform a laparoscopy to make sure that what is seen on the ultrasound is a fibroid. This often happens if the ovaries can't be clearly seen, because the suspected fibroid might really be an ovarian cyst or a cancerous growth. Another reason your doctor may want to do a laparotomy is when a fibroid suddenly grows very quickly. This is to rule out the possibility that the fibroid might be a cancerous tumour.

The medical approach

There are three main options for the management of fibroids:

- Observation.
- Drugs to reduce the size of fibroids. These drugs have two different effects, but the overall aim is to reduce the level of oestrogen. The drugs used are Danazol, to boost androgens and suppress oestrogens; and GnRH agonists, which induce a medical menopause.

When you stop using the GnRH agonists, the fibroids can grow back — sometimes within two or three weeks. They are usually only used prior to surgical removal.

- Surgical removal of the fibroid, called a myomectomy or, more commonly, a hysterectomy, the removal of the uterus (explained under Surgery in The Medical Approach chapter).

Natural therapies

Regulate excessive bleeding

It is often surprisingly easy to reduce the excessive bleeding caused by fibroids and this may be all that you want, especially if you have passed your childbearing years, your fibroids are small, or you are against surgery.

You may be prescribed any of the herbs favoured for the treatment of the heavy bleeding. Good ones for fibroids are *Alchemilla vulgaris* (ladies mantle), *Geranium maculatum* (cranesbill), *Equisetum arvense*, *Achillea millefolium*, *Tienchi ginseng*, *Hydrastis canadensis*, and *Capsella bursa-pastoris* (shepherd's purse). Astringent herbs are usually combined with one or more of the uterine tonic herbs to improve the uterine tone and try to normalise uterine function.

Getting the herbal mix right requires training and experience. A herbalist might prescribe herbs which affect uterine tone and regulate uterine bleeding — the astringents and uterine tonics; as well as herbs to treat the liver, and help to clear excess oestrogen.

Regulate relative oestrogen excess

It is important to control relative oestrogen excess because otherwise you might just keep growing multiple fibroids. And if you have them surgically removed without addressing the hormone situation, more might grow. An outline of the types of treatments and lifestyle changes you will need are in the section on too much oestrogen in the Usual Suspects chapter, page 33.

Reducing fibroid size

Considering the number of women who develop fibroids, the research on treatment isn't up to scratch. In one of the few trials using herbs to treat fibroids, the herbs *Paeonia lactiflora* and *P. suffruticosa*, *Poria cocos*, *Cinnamomum cassia* and *Prunus persica* were given to women with uterine fibroids. Ninety per cent of the women experienced an improvement of their symptoms and in 60 per cent of the cases, the fibroids got smaller.

Other herbs prescribed to treat fibroids and reduce their size include *Calendula officinalis*, *Thuja occiden-talis*, *Ruta graveolens* and *Tunera diffusa*. Vitamin E is believed to reduce fibroid size, but the reasons for this are unclear.

Self care

Follow all of the hints outlined in the section on too much oestrogen in the chapter called The Usual Suspects (pages 34–6).

Erratic Bleeding

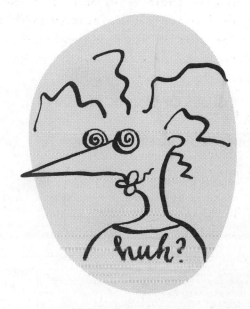

The most common cause of erratic bleeding is dysfunctional uterine bleeding — DUB for short — which is caused by erratic messages from the hypothalamus and pituitary in the brain to the ovary (we'll explain all about DUB in a minute). This is not a serious complaint in most cases, but a number of other conditions that also cause erratic bleeding can be. Hence we start with a warning and a description of those. The short, take-home message is: You must see your doctor if you have erratic bleeding or bleeding between periods, especially when:

· it's not part of your usual cycle;

- you're 40 or older;
- it happens after any kind of sex.

Any vaginal bleeding after menopause must be investigated immediately by a doctor no matter how small, because it could be uterine cancer. Other causes of post-menopausal bleeding might be polyps or lesions on the cervix.

COMMON CAUSES OF ERRATIC BLEEDING

Dysfunctional Uterine Bleeding see page 106

Endometrial hyperplasia
The endometrial cells are excessively stimulated by prolonged exposure to too much oestrogen in relation to progesterone. Not ovulating (ovulation guarantees the presence of progesterone) is the usual cause. Endometrial hyperplasia is diagnosed by examining a tissue sample under a microscope. The tissue is collected during a hysteroscopy or dilatation and curettage (D&C) surgery. (They are fully described under Surgery in The Medical Approach chapter.) The condition can lead to endometrial cancer if untreated. Common symptoms are irregular bleeding, spotting, and/or heavy, persistent flow.

Uterine cancer
Cancer of the uterus (commonly of the endometrium) is more likely over age 40. Symptoms include abnormal or recurrent bleeding between periods, after sex or after the

menopause. Over 40, these symptoms, however scant or fleeting, should always be investigated.

Polyps
A polyp is an overgrowth of tissue, which is attached by a stem or pedicle. They can happen in the cervix and endometrium. The cells of the polyp are often normal, but can bleed easily. They often bleed after sex or examination by a doctor. Women over 40 with cervical polyps may also have endometrial polyps.

Abnormalities of the cervix
Abnormalities of the cervix can cause bleeding and/or pain.

Cervical eversion/ectropion
If the cells which normally line the cervical canal grow down and onto the outer areas of the cervix, the 'overflow' is called a cervical ectropion or eversion. These cells are not as tough as the usual cells of the cervix and usually bleed more easily, especially on contact.

Cervical dysplasia and cancer
Both cervical cancer and dysplasia are detected with a Pap smear. Cervical dysplasia is a 'pre-cancerous condition' which does NOT mean you will automatically get cancer. It means the cells are changing and may eventually become cancerous if left untreated. Dysplasia is more common between 30 and 40 years old; cervical cancer is more common in the fifties. Both conditions cause few symptoms, and by the time bleeding has developed, the

condition can be quite advanced. Regular Pap tests, once a year in young and sexually active women, once every two years for others, can avoid this.

Cervicitis

This is inflammation of the cells of the cervix, usually from chronic infection. Vaginal discharge is a common symptom which may be accompanied by pain or contain brownish blood and have a yukky smell.

Conditions affecting the ovaries

Conditions affecting the ovaries don't always show up as a result of investigating abnormal bleeding. Usually pain is the initial symptom.

Ovarian cysts

Ovarian cysts are sacs of fluid in the ovary. They may be a consequence of the normal ovarian cycle. They may be benign or more rarely, cancerous. Over the age of 45, one in three ovarian cysts are malignant, and must be removed quick smart. Some cysts can interfere with the regularity of the period.

Ovulation

Some women experience spotting with pain (would you believe doctors call this mittelschmerz) at the time of normal ovulation. The bleeding is presumed to be caused by the oestrogen changes at mid-cycle, but is relatively rare and should be investigated.

Hormonal contraceptives

The combined (oestrogen and progesterone) Pill; the sequential Pill (Pills containing oestrogen and progesterone varied throughout the cycle); the Mini Pill (progesterone only) and Depo-Provera (an injection of slowly absorbed progesterone) can all be associated with abnormal bleeding patterns.

Malnutrition or excess weight loss

This may be due to severe illness, unavailable food, inadequate food, eating disorders or excessive exercise. Usually periods stop, although rarely heavier periods may be the result.

Pregnancy

Placental problems during pregnancy

- Bleeding caused by abnormal development of the placenta and/or a foetus.
- Bleeding related to a normally developing placenta, which is in the wrong place. This is called a 'placenta praevia'.
- Bleeding caused by normal placenta dislodging from the uterine wall too early. This is an 'accidental haemorrhage' and is very painful.

Hydatidiform mole

This results from a malformed foetus, and the pregnancy cannot continue. The tissue secretes large amounts of a hormone which usually causes severe 'morning sickness'. Often heavy bleeding starts about 10-12 weeks into the pregnancy, but will generally continue until all the mole is expelled. As this tissue can become cancerous, a D&C is recommended to remove all the tissue, and hormones are monitored for a year.

Ectopic pregnancy

An ectopic pregnancy is one which has started to develop outside the uterus. The embryo may be in the Fallopian tube, within the fimbriae of the ovary, or in the pelvic cavity. Ectopic pregnancies do not develop normally because there is no endometrium to sustain the developing placenta. If the pregnancy develops in the tube, the tube can rupture. This is dangerous and usually requires emergency surgery.

DYSFUNCTIONAL UTERINE BLEEDING (DUB)

What is dysfunctional uterine bleeding?

DUB isn't caused by an underlying disease: it's one of those disorders where there is a problem with the hormone balance. Basically what happens is the hormone control centre – the hypothalamus and pituitary glands situated in the brain – sends the wrong messages to the ovary, which in turn produces the wrong levels of oestrogen and progesterone. Progesterone in particular is important for the normal development of the lining in the uterus. When there is little or no progesterone, the endometrium does not develop and shed as it would during a normal cycle. Instead it tends either to break away in bits and pieces, causing spotting or erratic and long periods, or to come away in a rush, causing the flooding or very heavy periods seen with DUB. (See pages 108–9 for more info.)

Symptoms

Basically DUB can cause just about any irregularity of the menstrual cycle. Below, we describe some of the common erratic bleeding patterns.

Spotting or bleeding between periods

The fancy name for unscheduled bleeding is metror-rhagia, pronounced metro-rah-jee-ar. It means bleeding at times other than the period. Sometimes it's called inter-menstrual bleeding or threshold bleeding. The bleeding often happens at the time of ovulation, although it may happen at any time during the cycle.

This type of bleeding might be very slight and is then usually referred to as 'spotting' — so named for the effect it has on your undies gusset. Spotting might occur just before or after the period, or at any time during the cycle. It's the slight bleeding that can be most suggestive of cancer or other serious problems, many of which must be treated early. Spotting after sex can be the big warning sign of cancerous lesions of the uterus or cervix. So, off to the doctor with you and no hiding behind the couch.

Heavier bleeding between periods is often caused by DUB — but it could be caused by cancer of the cervix or uterus, and until that possibility has been investigated and eliminated as the cause, no treatment should be under-taken. It is vital that you don't just take a drug or herbs to stop bleeding without knowing exactly what is going on.

Irregular periods

When a woman has DUB the period can happen at intervals of less than 21 days, and is called polymenorrhoea (pronounced polly-men-oh-rear). Causes again are usually misbehaviour of the hypothalamic-pituitary unit or the ovary. Often, the problem is to do with ovulation happening too early. On the other hand, ovulation might stop for a time and the cycle might become too long – known as oligomenorrhoea.

Too often and too heavy

Polymenorrhagia (pronounced polly-men-o-rah-jee-ar) is a combination of menorrhagia (heavy periods) and polymenorrhoea (too many periods) and can also be a problem if you have DUB. Thank God it doesn't include another complaint as well or we'd be here all day trying to spell it, let alone pronounce it.

Causes

In many cases of DUB, ovulation is abnormal, or fails entirely. This leads to an imbalance in the hormones – oestrogen is still pumping out, but progesterone production is either far too low or gone altogether. This results in the 'unopposed' oestrogen overstimulating the endometrium (uterus lining) and leads to the characteristic bleeding patterns – an erratic cycle, no obvious signs of ovulation, and irregular or prolonged episodes of bleeding.

In the normal course of events, oestrogen is 'opposed' by the presence of progesterone. The progesterone production and withdrawal maintains the regularity of the endometrial shedding (and therefore the period). When you don't ovulate (or progesterone production is too low), oestrogen continues to stimulate the endometrial cells which grow and thicken. But the absence of progesterone means that the endometrium does not develop the usual structural features of the secretory phase, including special tiny blood vessels to nourish the endometrium and control blood loss once the period starts.

Without the development of these blood vessels, circulation throughout the thickened endometrium eventually fails; and the tissue becomes fragile and starts to break down. This does not happen uniformly throughout the endometrium — some bits are shed while others remain intact, resulting in the spotting and erratic blood loss.

At the same time, the hormonal imbalance may lead to disordered prostaglandins. In a normal cycle, the body slows the blood loss using prostaglandins to increase uterine tone and cause spasm of the spiral arterioles. Without these, you can get really heavy bleeding. This type of DUB is most common when regular ovulation is at its most fragile: among teenagers who have just started to get periods, and around the menopause. It can also be a feature of any condition where ovulation doesn't happen, such as thyroid disease, androgen excess, and obesity. It's often caused by stress.

Diagnosis

The diagnosis of DUB is a diagnosis of exclusion, so other conditions must be eliminated as the cause of bleeding. Signs and symptoms highly suggestive of DUB are:

- Age. Women who are establishing their normal cyclical pattern in the first few years of their period, and women whose cycles are slowing down around menopause are more likely to develop DUB.

- Normal uterine size and normal cervix. Because spotting can also be a feature of something wrong with the cervix, a healthy cervix means the spotting is more likely to be DUB. The uterus can get bigger and change shape if you have fibroids or adenomyosis, both common causes of heavy periods.

- A recent history of persistent or severe stress. Because of its effect on the hypothalamic-pituitary function, stress can stop ovulation or disrupt progesterone production.

- A reliable negative pregnancy test. Pregnancy-related bleeding is the most common cause of abnormal period patterns.

- No pain during a vaginal examination or an abdominal palpation by a doctor. Pelvic inflammatory disease and endometriosis are two conditions which can cause symptoms similar to DUB, but they both usually cause pain during an examination.

- A normal ultrasound. Ultrasounds will detect any abnormal thickening of the endometrium which could indicate endometrial hyperplasia; or any growths in the uterus such as polyps.

The medical approach

A synthetic progesterone drug, usually Provera or Primulut, is used to try to interrupt the abnormal hormonal pattern and regulate the cycle. The use of a diagnostic curette (D&C) or hysteroscopy on older women to determine whether the bleeding is caused by endometrial hyperplasia or cancer has been superseded by the use of the ultrasound. There's detailed info on the drugs and surgery in the Medical Approach chapter.

Natural therapies

The treatment of DUB aims to re-establish ovulation, support the luteal phase of the cycle, treat stress where appropriate, and use any or all of the treatments necessary to control bleeding. (There's a list of these on page 99 in the section on regulating excessive bleeding associated with fibroids.)

Around the time of the first period, erratic cycles are so common that it's usually thought of as being physiological — in other words, a normal feature. So young women with dysfunctional bleeding patterns don't usually require any treatment unless the bleeding is particularly severe and causing other problems. Herbal remedies which are appropriate for erratic bleeding experienced around this time are *Achillea millefolium* (yarrow), *Equisetum arvense* (horsetail), *Rubus idaeus* (raspberry leaves) and *Alchemilla vulgaris* (ladies mantle).

Herbs to re-establish ovulation

In order to re-establish ovulation, it is first necessary to find out why it went away. This may be related to the life stage — around menopause or the first period; or ovulation may temporarily stop because of stress, overexercising, low body weight or a poor diet. Sometimes the exact cause is unknown. (If a doctor ever says to you: 'The reason for your problem is idiopathic', don't faint. Idiopathic is just the doctor's word for 'There's no scientific reason for what's causing this'.)

Not ovulating can be caused by complex hormonal irregularities related to the endocrinal glands. These conditions are treated by fixing any abnormal function of the other glands, such as the thyroid or the adrenal gland; or addressing a major disruption in ovarian function like polycystic ovaries; or treating the abnormal activity of the hypothalamic–pituitary unit, such as hyperprolactinaemia.

The main herb for DUB is *Vitex agnus castus*. This herb improves ovulation rates and is generally prescribed for any problem in the luteal phase of the cycle associated with progesterone. It is easy to cause unwanted problems by taking *Vitex* without the supervision of a herbalist because you have to be careful with the dose, the time of day it's taken, when it's started and how long you stay on it. Get professional advice before taking this herb. A herb with similar action is *Paeonia lactiflora*, but it is even more difficult to self prescribe and so you'll need help with this one too.

'Female tonic' herbs are used to re-establish normal bleeding patterns. These herbs may interact with the hypothalamus or the pituitary to re-start ovulation. The most important of these are *Tribulus terrestris*, *Aletris farinosa*, *Dioscorea villosa* and *Trillium erectum*.

Trillium erectum (beth root) contains hormone-like plant substances called diosgenins, which seem to help regulate both the blood flow and the hormone balance. Another herb, *Alchemilla vulgaris* has similar effects. These uterine tonic herbs are considered to be 'specific' to the treatment of DUB, which is caused by not ovulating, and can regulate both cycle length and period flow within one to three cycles.

The advice given under the section on PMS A is generally useful for DUB because it aims to improve the symptoms associated with progesterone deficiency.

Self care

- Read the section on not enough progesterone in the Usual Suspects chapter, page 38. The advice for PMS A on pages 68–9 may be suggested by your practitioner.
- Minimise stress. Apart from anything else, erratic and heavy bleeding is stressful in itself and the worry caused by having the symptoms may feed into the stress cycle and worsen the symptoms. Stress management hints are also included on pages 45–6.

Not Getting Your Period

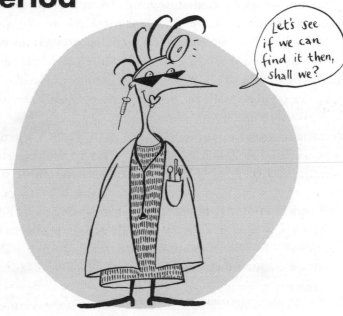

Let's see if we can find it then, shall we?

Even though we might make a joke about the unbounded joy of not having to bother with periods, the 'convenience' needs to be weighed against the need to find out the cause of the missing period. If you've already started your periods and you then stop for more than six months, you may be told you have amenorrhoea (pronounced ay-men-oh-rear). Basically it just means stopped periods, or no periods. A range of hormonal, physical and metabolic conditions, including Polycystic Ovarian Syndrome

(PCOS), which we'll explain in a minute, can cause the period to stop.

Needless to say, it is absolutely vital that treatment should only proceed after identifying the underlying problem. Don't let anyone 'treat' you to bring your period back without knowing why it went away.

PCOS can also cause primary amenorrhoea, where you haven't had your first period by 17.

LESS COMMON CAUSES OF STOPPED PERIODS

Not getting your first period can be caused by a number of congenital and hormonal factors. In extremely rare cases, a young woman might not have a uterus or have another congenital abnormality — maybe a blockage in the vagina which stops the blood flow. There are a few hormonal irregularities that can delay or stop the first period.

In many cases, there is no major physical problem, the onset of puberty has simply been delayed, and periods will come along in their own time. Delayed onset of puberty, however, is a diagnosis of exclusion, and most doctors will want to make absolutely sure there's nothing else the matter. First they check to see whether you have all systems go on the oestrogen front.

If you have any development in the bosoms department, it means that either your ovaries are making oestrogen, or the body is converting androgens to oestrogens in the fat tissues. Full breast development only happens when your ovaries are making oestrogen, so how developed your breasts are (this has nothing to do with actual size) gives important clues to the causes of the lack of period.

The next step is an ultrasound to make sure you have a uterus and all the right accessories. (See Screening in the Medical Approach chapter.)If there's still no problem, the next step is to take blood tests to see if there's a hormone problem. Usually the levels of follicle stimulating hormone (FSH), luteinising hormone (LH), and prolactin (the breast-related hormone) are checked. Normal levels of all three are seen in delayed puberty; while a high LH with a low FSH is seen in polycystic ovarian disease. Other possible causes are a high prolactin level, usually indicating a pituitary tumour called a prolactinoma, or a high FSH and LH indicating a possible 'resistant ovary syndrome'.

COMMON CAUSES OF STOPPED PERIODS (SECONDARY AMENORRHOEA)

Polycystic Ovarian Syndrome (PCOS), see page 118

Hypothalamus problems
The hypothalamus, a hormone secreting gland in the brain, usually secretes gonadotrophin releasing hormone (GnRH) in pulses, but a number of conditions can interfere, including:
Stress, including travel, can stop periods. The oestrogen levels are in the lower range and often ovulation doesn't happen.

Weight loss Periods can stop if the body fat content drops below 15–20 per cent. (See Being Underweight in the Usual Suspects section). Common causes are not eating properly, anorexia nervosa and serious illness.

Overexercise GnRH is badly affected by prolonged and rigorous exercise, and this can stop periods.

Severe chronic illness Chronic renal or liver failure, and other severe or prolonged illnesses can stop periods because of their effect on the hypothalamus.

Drugs Some prescribed and illegal drugs can interfere with hormones.

Post-pill amenorrhoea About 80 per cent of women get a period within three months of stopping the Pill, but about 1 per cent will experience long-term post-Pill absent periods. Some of these women have pre-existing conditions, such as polycystic ovarian syndrome, which haven't been noticed while the Pill caused regular 'periods'.

Not ovulating

A number of conditions can lead to prolonged dysfunction of the ovaries and no periods.

Breastfeeding is initially triggered by high prolactin levels which can stop ovulation and periods. The effect usually lasts a few months — but breastfeeding is not a reliable contraceptive.

Some **thyroid conditions** and a handful of other medical causes.

POLYCYSTIC OVARIAN SYNDROME (PCOS)

Here's the confusing part: firstly there's a condition called polycystic ovaries (PCO), which literally means there are too many cysts in the ovary or ovaries. And then there's this whole other thing called polycystic ovarian syndrome (PCOS). This is a much more complicated condition associated with the production of high levels of androgens (male hormones) and irregular ovulation which increase the tendency to develop symptoms such as excess hair growth, acne, blood sugar abnormalities, weight gain and infertility, in conjunction with the multiple ovarian cysts. The severity and presence of these symptoms vary greatly between women, but together they make up the syndrome known as PCOS.

According to ultrasound examinations, up to one in five women have multiple ovarian cysts (PCO). Of these women, about one quarter will *not* develop the additional hormonal abnormalities that indicate they have PCOS and may only do so in the presence of an appropriate trigger such as weight gain. So while some of them have both normal cycles and periods and experience no problems, others may not menstruate at all, may stop menstruating, or could develop a range of menstrual irregularities such as irregular cycles and/or abnormally light periods.

As you can imagine, there is a fair bit of confusion about the two terms because many writers, doctors and natural therapists do not differentiate between polycystic ovaries and polycystic ovarian syndrome. To sum up, anyone with many 'simple' cysts on their ovaries has polycystic ovaries. Those who have lots of cysts on their ovaries and hormonal abnormalities have polycystic ovarian syndrome (PCOS).

To add further confusion, some women develop all or some of the endocrine signs associated with PCOS (hirsutism, acne, weight gain, irregular periods or infertility) but do not have multiple ovarian cysts. There is some debate over whether these women have true PCOS or whether they have an entirely different complaint. From a treatment point of view, however, there is no difference between these women and those who have PCOS with ovarian cysts. This section deals only with PCOS. (PCOS and the less frequently used term, PCOD (polycystic ovarian disease) are interchangeable terms.)

Making a diagnosis of PCOS is further complicated because these symptoms just mentioned can also happen to people who don't have PCOS at all. Women with similar symptoms might have something else entirely, like a misbehaving thyroid gland.

Diagnosis
PCOS is usually suspected if you have developed irregular periods or stopped periods, you're carrying around extra weight, can't seem to get pregnant and have more facial hair than usual — 'male-pattern' hair growth. An ultrasound of the ovaries will usually detect multiple cysts. Before a firm diagnosis of PCOS can be made, all of the other possible types of endocrine abnormalities need to be excluded as causes. This involves a physical examination and blood tests in addition to the ultrasound. (More ultrasound info is under Screening in The Medical Approach chapter.)

Causes

A number of important factors seem to make a contribution to the development of PCOS. These may be different for individual women, and might be associated with early life changes such as childhood obesity or maternal gestational diabetes. Putting on extra weight or having insulin resistance can trigger hormonal changes that seems to be able to kick symptom-free simple cysts into a full-on case of PCOS. It has been suggested that other endocrine glands like the ovary, the adrenal glands or the thyroid might also be implicated in leading to PCOS in some women. PCOS may also be inherited. Around 40 per cent of the women in families with PCOS will have the condition, but not all of them will develop symptoms.

It is not clear which of these possible hormonal problems is the trigger for PCOS becoming evident in the first place. However, once these hormonal changes start the cycle of PCOS, they can eventually give rise to a 'hormonal steady state', devoid of the usual monthly fluctuations typical of the female menstrual cycle. In other words, the hormonal abnormalities become 'locked in' and cause the amenorrhoea, lack of ovulation or irregular menstrual bleeding seen in up to 90 per cent of women with PCOS.

Androgen excess

Androgens, made in the ovaries and the adrenal glands, usually circulate in small amounts in the blood of all women without causing any symptoms.

If you've got PCOS, however, you've got too many male hormones — not as many as blokes have, but enough to cause a hormone imbalance and the symptoms of PCOS. (There's more info on androgen excess later in this chapter.)

Abnormal ovarian function

Women with PCOS have been found to have low levels of ovarian oestrogen (oestradiol) and high levels of ovarian androgens, indicating that the problem starts in the ovary (basically the girly hormones are being outflanked by the blokey hormones.) The androgens produced within the follicle (the bit that makes the egg) seem to prevent ovulation and normal egg development. The end result is that the eggs become cysts instead, so that's why ovulation doesn't happen. Some women with PCOS have one ovary that's normal and one that's polycystic.

The adrenal glands

It may be that the adrenal glands are the source of the excess androgens and not the ovaries. Once the adrenal glands start pumping out too many androgens, they are then faithfully converted to oestrone by the fatty tissue. These high, constant oestrone levels suppress the egg-making follicular hormone, and encourage too much luteinising hormone which in turn tells the body to make even more androgens — and so on in a vicious circle.

Insulin resistance

Insulin resistance occurs when insulin cannot transport glucose into cells as it should. It is often seen in conjunction with PCOS. This is thought to be because insulin resistance over-stimulates the activity of the adrenal glands which then produce too many androgens and cause the events explained above. Although it was once believed that insulin resistance only occurred in association with obesity, it has now been shown that both obese and non-obese women with PCOS can develop insulin resistance. Insulin resistance is described in more detail in the Natural Therapies chapter on page 189.

Excess weight gain
Various bits of the body convert androgens into an oestrogen called oestrone by a process called aromatisation — not to be confused with lighting smelly candles and having a lavender bubble bath. One of the parts of the body which aromatises is fatty tissue. So if you are overweight, there are more fatty tissues converting androgen into more and more oestrone. This maintains really high levels of oestrogen in the body all month long, instead of the natural cycle causing the normal ups and downs of oestrogen.

Some women can control the severity of PCOS and the regularity of their menstrual cycle by reducing their overall weight. If you have PCOS you'll probably take to being thin better than other women. It is likely you may be able to maintain your bone density even when your Body Mass Index (BMI) is low, and continue to ovulate (or start to) when you're thin. Women with 'normal' ovaries function best in the reproductive department and maintain bone density when they carry more weight and their BMI is in the middle of the range. (See the section on the BMI in The Usual Suspects for how to calculate your BMI.)

Sex hormone binding globulin
High levels of androgen and obesity also suppress the sex hormone binding globulin (SHBG), a protein which transports both oestrogen and testosterone around the body. Normally, the SHBG 'babysits' the body's testosterone.

When SHBG levels drop, the testosterone runs wild, causing acne and male-pattern hair growth.

Signs and symptoms
- About half of women with PCOS will not have periods.
- Nearly a third have abnormal bleeding patterns.
- Only about 10 per cent have regular period cycles.
- PCOS is the most common cause of not ovulating: about 75 per cent of women with PCOS develop infertility (if you don't make the eggs, you can't get them fertilised).
- About 60 per cent of women with PCOS have excess body hair.
- Around 40 per cent are overweight.
- About 20 per cent develop 'male' characteristics such as a deeper voice and changes in body shape.
- About 15 per cent have the basal body temperature changes which indicate ovulation.

The medical approach
The first thing to know about PCOS is that you may need no treatment at all. If symptoms are mild with only a

slightly irregular cycle, following a sensible diet, maintaining body weight in the normal range and exercising regularly may be all that's needed. However, if fertility, excess hair growth or acne is a problem, or if cycles are very intermittent or have stopped completely then the following advice along with a visit to a health care practitioner skilled in this area will be useful.

Regulate the cycle
If periods have stopped, periods should be brought about to protect the endometrium from too much cell build-up which can eventually become cancerous — it's the endometrium which bleeds away during a period. Doctors prescribe cyclic hormones like the Pill, or small doses of progesterone for seven to ten days each month after which the 'period' will come on. The progesterone, either taken alone or in the Pill, initiates changes in the endometrium which are similar to those in the normal cycle. (There's more on these drugs in The Medical Approach chapter.)

Induce ovulation with drugs
Fertility drugs, such as Clomid, are used if you want to get pregnant. Side effects and ethical issues, such as multiple births and embryo selection, should be discussed with your doctor. Metformin (Glucophage), a drug used for insulin resistance and diabetes, is also sometimes prescribed to improve fertility.

Reduce unwanted hair growth
The most common drugs prescribed are Androcur (cyproterone acetate) or the Pill called Diane (can you BELIEVE

manufacturers called a pill Diane? What are they thinking? Do you reckon there's a prostate drug called Bruce, for God's sake?) The hair often grows back when the person stops the drug. Another common drug is Aldactone, which was originally used for high blood pressure. It also blocks the effects of androgens.

Natural therapies

The tendency to develop PCOS cannot be 'cured' but hormones can be regulated so that symptoms are minimised. If you have bad PCOS, natural remedies may not be strong enough to control your feral hormones. Combining natural remedies and drugs might be more useful, especially when there is serious risk of endometrial change or severe masculinising effects from androgens. Natural therapists share the same aims as the medical approach, using different means. The emphasis of natural treatments will depend on the combination of the symptoms and your idea of a successful outcome.

Regulate the cycle

The most important herbs for cycle regulation are *Glycyrrhiza glabra* (liquorice) and *Paeonia lactiflora* (peony):

Glycyrrhiza glabra (liquorice)
Compounds in liquorice slow down the conversion of weak androgens into stronger ones in the ovary and in the hair follicle. This means that liquorice can be used to treat hirsutism by slowing the conversion of weaker androgens into the more active androgen testosterone.

125 **?**

In addition, liquorice also slows down ovarian production of androgens, as well as being able to calm down the overactivity of the adrenal glands that is caused by insulin resistance. So, all in all, it's pretty important for PCOS and excess androgens.

Paeonia lactiflora (peony)

Peony is thought to act directly on the ovary to reduce the production of the androgens. It increases the activity of aromatase which promotes the synthesis of oestradiol from testosterone. Peony-containing formulas may also improve progesterone levels by normalising ovarian function when the activity of aromatase is inhibited.

Liquorice and peony combination

Liquorice and peony are almost always prescribed together as most of the research on the herbal treatment of PCOS has been done on this combination. These herbs should be prescribed by a practitioner experienced in the treatment of PCOS.

Liquorice can cause a number of serious side effects. These include low blood potassium, combined with high blood sodium and fluid retention. This can cause high blood pressure and heart problems. Again we stress that liquorice should only be prescribed by a qualified herbalist and under close supervision.

Relatively small doses over a long period are used for PCOS, however, the following recommendations are necessary:

- a diet high in potassium and low in sodium

- blood pressure surveillance increased with increasing duration of use
- serum potassium levels may need to be monitored
- decoctions of *Taraxacum officinale* leaf can be used to reduce the risk of low blood potassium levels and hypertension.

Liquorice should not be prescribed at the same time as *spironolactone* (Aldactone), a common anti-androgenic and anti-hypertensive drug.

Reduce the risk of endometrial cancer

For the endometrium to be adequately protected, you need regular periods.

These intervals vary depending on your weight and age. If you're within the normal weight range, and aged 35 or under, you should have at least three periods every year. Older women, particularly if they're overweight, should have at least six a year (until the menopause, obviously).

Obese women, who are likely to have more problems with PCOS, should be having a period each month if they can. For this reason, the Pill may be your best treatment option to protect the endometrium if you're obese and at increased risk of endometrial hyperplasia or cancer.

Herbs which can bring on periods should only be prescribed by a qualified herbalist. The safest way to bring on a period is to stimulate ovulation (see below).

Stimulate ovulation to regulate the cycle

Some herbs are believed to be able to normalise ovulation, and can be prescribed by a professional herbalist with specific experience in this area. *Tribulus terrestris* is a beauty as it is also used in infertility. Another useful herb is *Paeonia lactiflora*. In combination with *Glycyrrhiza glabra* (liquorice) it has been shown to improve ovulation rates and thus assist fertility. *Cimicifuga racemosa*, best known for use against menopausal symptoms, also gets the menstrual cycle into gear because of its effect on luteinising hormone (LH). It is particularly useful for PCOS when used with hops and peony.

The other helpful group of herbs are the 'female tonic' herbs. This group are usually 'oestrogenic' and contain phyto-oestrogens or steroidal saponins. They exert a much weaker effect than oestrogen and may kick-start ovulation by increasing the levels of follicle stimulating hormone (FSH).

Included in this group are *Dioscorea villosa* and *Aletris farinosa*. *Vitex agnus castus* should be cautiously prescribed for this condition because although it stimulates ovulation, it may increase luteinising hormone which you definitely don't need.

Reduce unwanted hair growth or acne

Male-pattern hair growth or acne seen in PCOS is caused by androgens and can be difficult to control with herbs or other natural methods. The *Smilax* species (sarsaparilla) and *Turnera aphrodisiaca* (damiana) seem to block the effects of androgens by competitive inhibition, but drugs are faster and more reliable. When excess hair growth or acne is a serious problem, drugs first, followed by herbal remedies for maintenance, can be the best combo.

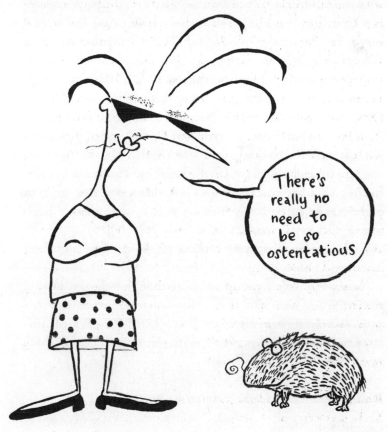

Hairy problems

Another method is to increase the rate at which androgens are converted by the body to oestrogens. Peony and liquorice combination (see page 126), a formula used in traditional Chinese medicine, can be successful.

The adrenal gland contribution to androgens may be modified by adaptogen herbs including *Eleuthrococcus senticosus* (Siberian ginseng) and *Panax ginseng* (Korean ginseng). The nervines, a group of herbs used to moderate the effects of stress (see Stress in the Usual Suspects chapter for details), may also be helpful. *Humulus lupulus* (hops) which is a nervine and has the additional benefit of lowering luteinising hormone is an important herb for PCOS.

When excess hair growth is the primary concern, treatment must be continued for many months, and in some cases indefinitely. It is important that the chosen herbal remedies are considered safe for long-term administration. It is vital that you work with a trained herbalist with a speciality in this area, and (all together now) don't self-prescribe.

Treating the accompanying complaints

Luteinising hormone
Too much luteinising hormone (LH) causes too much androgen around the place, and when LH levels fall, so do androgens. Three herbs have a direct impact on luteinising hormone: *Cimicifuga racemosa* (black cohosh), *Humulus lupulus* (hops), and *Lycopus virginiana* (bugleweed). Hops and black cohosh are especially good when stress and nervous tension accompany PCOS. Both seem

also to inhibit the effect of oestrogen. *Lycopus virginiana* is usually given to treat hyperthyroidism, but will also reduce the levels of LH as well as follicle stimulating hormone (FSH). It should only be taken short term, and if you're trying to ovulate properly again. Remember, don't self-prescribe.

Blood sugar abnormalities

Women with PCOS are prone to blood sugar abnormalities which develop as a result of obesity and insulin resistance as described earlier. The priority is to lose weight and help the insulin to get into the cells. The nutrients which help are magnesium, zinc (info pages on these are under Minerals in the Self Care chapter) and manganese and chromium. Herbs you may be prescribed include *Gymnema sylvestra* (gymnema), *Galagea officinalis* (goat's rue), *Trigonella foenum-graecum* (fenugreek), and the bitters. Insulin resistance responds to dietary changes and the guidelines can be found on pages 190–1.

Phyto-oestrogens and fibre have a beneficial effect on blood sugar abnormalities and also reduce the severity of symptoms associated with androgen excess by making the androgens less biologically available. They are described in more detail in the section on plant oestrogens on page 194.

Regulating the blood lipid levels

About three-quarters of women with PCOS have blood fats ('lipids') abnormalities. The general principles of blood fats regulation involve eating stuff like the bitter herbs, high-fibre foods, and phyto-oestrogens (legumes like lentils and soya products), and reducing animal fats. More on Bad Fats and Good Fats in the 20 Good-Eating Hints in the Self Care chapter.

The Medical Approach

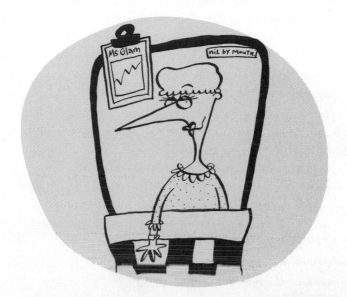

CHOOSING AND WORKING WITH YOUR DOCTOR

Doctors to avoid include ones who smoke during a consultation, ones who want to do nude hokey-pokey with you as part of the diagnostic process, ones who say things like 'You leave it all up to me, dearie, you don't need to know the details', and doctors who insist that there is nothing valuable, under any circumstances, about natural therapies. Here's some ways to narrow the field:

- Find a sympathetic, smart, up-to-date general practitioner. Ask around, and then make up your own mind.

- Always ask if you don't understand something and keep asking until you do. It's not your failure to get it, it's the doctor's failure to make it clear for you.
- Take notes so you can review them afterwards. If you are being asked to absorb a lot of information at once, especially for the first time, you can walk out with your head in a fog, remembering afterwards only the bit where you think the doctor said, 'I'm afraid you've got myxomatosis'.
- First consultations with a specialist are usually half an hour, to allow the doctor to fully explore your medical history. Follow-up consultations will vary.
- Get a second opinion, or extra opinions, if you are unsure or unhappy with any recommendation by a general practitioner, specialist or surgeon.
- Always tell the doctor anything you think is relevant to your condition. This definitely includes other medications, herbs or supplements like vitamins you may be taking.
- Always follow the instructions on medicine exactly. Just because 10 milligrams makes you feel better, it doesn't mean 20 milligrams will be twice as good.
- When choosing a specialist for your particular problem, do as much research as you can about their experience, expertise and manner. Don't be afraid to try a few out before you decide.
- Find out if your surgeon is experienced in the latest specialised techniques, or is more of an all-round gynaecologist. For complicated conditions, find a doctor who specialises in your problem.

- If you have surgery, the surgeon may visit you after the operation while you are still groggy. You may not remember the surgeon's report later. To be fully informed about what happened during your operation, and the implications for the future, get somebody to take notes for you then, organise a telephone call for a better time, or insist on an appointment as soon as you're up.
- Always tell the practitioner if you are pregnant, trying to get pregnant, wouldn't mind getting pregnant or are not perfectly strict with contraception.

SCREENING

Any full check-up will involve a breast examination, a Pap test, a pelvic examination, and blood tests which are taken by the doctor or nurse and analysed in a pathology lab. Any vaginal bleeding after menopause must be investigated immediately by a doctor no matter how small, because it could be uterine cancer. Other causes of post-menopausal bleeding might be polyps or lesions on the cervix.

Here's what to expect and when to request a particular test:

Pelvic examinations

When

Every year. (And yes, you still need pelvic exams if you're a lesbian or celibate.)

Why

Pain on movement of the organs, or other tell-tale signs such as an organ feeling 'fixed' when it's supposed to be more mobile can indicate endometriosis, infection or adhesions. It can also detect unusual swellings, enlargement of the ovaries, uterine fibroids, pregnancy, cysts and tumours.

What

There are usually two stages to a pelvic 'exam'. Both are performed while you lie on your back on the couch in the doctor's office. It's okay to ask for a nurse to be there too. Here's the hard bit: with all that ferreting around going on down there you're supposed to relax. It's not exactly a calming experience, but it shouldn't hurt unless you tense up or there is something wrong. Sometimes the doctor will ask you to put your feet into 'stirrups'. (Try to resist the urge to say 'Giddy-up'.)

The doctor, wearing latex gloves over clean hands, will use a sterilised metal or plastic instrument called a speculum to very gently 'jack' open your vagina a little way so the doctor can look up the vagina and see the cervix. This is also a good time to have a Pap test, a case of 'While you're down there . . .

For the full pelvic exam, the doctor will put two fingers inside the vagina so the tips of the fingers are in the area at the top of the vagina between the cervix and the wall of the vagina. The doctor's other hand will be placed on your lower abdomen. The doctor very gently wiggles fingertips to jostle some of your organs to feel if they are the right size and shape. The uterus and ovaries can be felt between the hands and, if you are relaxed (well, relatively relaxed), it is fairly easy to tell whether they are in the normal place, the right size and can move easily.

Now go and buy yourself a cup of tea and some chocolate cake.

Pap test

When
Once every two years regardless of your sexual preference, unless your doctor advises you to have one more often.

Why
A Papanicolaou smear test (named after the doctor who invented it) is used to screen for changes to the cells on the cervix, which may proceed to cervical cancer if untreated.

What
See the speculum procedure above in the pelvic exam section. After this, the doctor inserts a tiny, skinny wooden or plastic spatula to gently scrape cells from the surface of the cervix. The cells are then smeared onto a glass slide, given a squirt with hair spray (well, it looks like hair spray but they reckon it's a fixative) and sent to a pathology lab for examination. (A new way of getting cells on the slide is being researched.) The procedure should be painless, but can be a little uncomfortable.

The cervical cells are examined under a microscope in a lab and graded according to the type of cells and whether they have undergone any changes. Pap tests can be inaccurate. When changes in cells are found in a Pap test, a colposcopy is often suggested. A colposcopy is a procedure in which a doctor looks up the vagina with a special telescope to see the cervix.

Breast checks

When
Every month after each period by you and an annual check by a doctor. Most women detect breast changes themselves. They know the 'normal' feel of their own breasts and are in a unique position to detect change and detect it early.

Why
You're looking for lumps or any changes in breast tissue. About 80 per cent of breast lumps are not cancerous, but even when a breast lump is caused by cancer, the earlier it is found, the better the outlook.

What
Breast examination involves two phases: visual and physical examination of the breast tissue. Do it after every period, and after menopause, once a month. You need to get to know intimately the feel of your breasts and report ANY changes to a doctor.

Now we could print a very involved chart here, but really, we'd prefer you went to the doctor and got a lesson in how to do it properly, because it's easy once you know how.

 138

To jog your memory, pick up a pamphlet while you're there or get one from the Women's Health Care Centre in your State or Territory (contact details are at the back of the book).

Mammogram

These are recommended every 2 years for women 50 and over, and more often for women who have had breast cancer or a strong possibility of developing breast cancer (for example a genetic predisposition). The mammogram operator will place one of your breasts on a metal plate and then bring another plate down on the top of your breast, squashing it as far as it can. A 'photograph' is then taken of the breast tissue, and that image will help a specialist identify areas of concern, including lumps that must be investigated. A mammogram will not be able to identify whether a lump is benign or malignant but can give the doctor a fairly clear idea of what type of lump has been discovered.

Ultrasound

This is a type of imaging using high-frequency sound waves to look at soft tissue structures in the breast or pelvis such as cysts or lumps. A sticky gel is smoothed over the skin and a small instrument, something similar to a computer mouse, is moved over the area. It doesn't hurt at all and is frequently used to tell whether a breast lump detected with a mammogram is a breast cancer or cyst, or whether you have fibroids or other cysts in the uterus or ovaries area.

Blood tests

Drink lots of water before you have blood taken, otherwise it can be harder to draw blood efficiently. Make sure you arrange a time to call or visit the doctor for the results.

HORMONE DRUGS

The bottom line is that many prescribed drugs have to be strong, and even toxic, to deal with the problem they target. The body can sometimes use a little help, either with something from a natural therapist to offset side effects, like a mineral or vitamin supplement, or by finding another drug or brand of drug that you tolerate better. Always talk to your doctor if you are having a rough time: there are often alternatives.

The Pill

There are many different types of oral contraceptives including Pills with variable oestrogen and progestogen levels (Triphasil and Triquilar), or those with the same levels throughout the cycle (Brevinor, Microgynon).

Some also contain androgen-blocking agents (Diane) and are used for acne and excessive male-pattern hair growth; some are progestogen-only Pills (the mini Pills such as Micronor and Microlut). A lot of factors need to be considered when prescribing the Pill. Each different brand or type of Pill can have its own effects on individuals. If you have any difficulties see a gynaecologist.

Good points

If taken properly, the Pill is pretty good contraception, but other good side effects may include reduced rates of ovarian and endometrial cancer, benign breast disease (not breast cancer), benign ovarian cysts, pelvic inflammatory disease, period pain, heavy periods and anaemia. Today's low-dose Pills are much safer than the earlier Pills which had much higher doses of hormones.

Bad points

The less jolly side effects of the Pill can include blood clots, stroke, and heart attack, especially for smokers. It can cause period changes such as breakthrough bleeding or spotting, and some women experience androgenic blokey hormone effects, including the weight gain and acne which are associated with the progestogen (synthetic progesterone) in the Pill.

A small number of women develop long-term loss of periods after coming off the Pill – estimated to be about 1 per cent after the first year.

Some women on the Pill also report an increase in mood swings, depression and loss of interest in sex. These symptoms are more common in the first couple of months of taking the Pill and may go away after that. Doctors usually advise taking one Pill for two months before trying a new brand of Pill which might be better tolerated.

Warnings in MIMS and the PP Guide (medical books which describe what drugs should be prescribed for, what the drugs do, and when they shouldn't be used) say that oestrogen can make fibroids get bigger. However, it has been shown that fibroids do not necessarily increase in size when women take the Pill, that periods become lighter and that blood-iron levels increase. If you have fibroids and you want to take the Pill, talk to a gynaecologist.

The Pill can cause increased pigmentation of the skin which is known as chloasma or melasma. This usually shows up in patchy, light brown areas on a pale-skinned face and becomes much darker with exposure to the sun. It is probably caused by oestrogen — it also can happen in pregnancy, or in women with high oestrogen levels. Stopping the Pill does not necessarily mean that it will go away completely, although it does tend to fade. Use sun block religiously, and you can lighten the pigmentation with safe skin creams or 'peels' that contain glycolic acid. Doctors sometimes recommend creams containing hydroquinone or acne medication.

Why it's used
Apart from its use as a contraceptive, the Pill is often prescribed for heavy periods. It usually reduces bleeding by thinning the endometrial lining. The Pill can also be used for period pain, especially when you need a contraceptive as well, or if prostaglandins-inhibitors like Naprogesic and Ponstan haven't worked for you. The Pill improves period pain about 90 per cent of the time because it stops ovulation and holds down the prostaglandins which cause muscle spasm.

The Pill improves PMS symptoms in some women, has no effect in others and makes some women worse. The Pill's control of some women's PMS is probably because it stops ovulation and balances the hormones.

Taking the Pill reduces the amount of period blood,

and so lowers the risk of developing endometriosis. The latest Pills have much lower levels of oestrogen and seem to reduce the amount of both normal endometrium and the amount of endometriosis. Even better results are found when the Pill is used continuously (without a break for 'periods') to create a pretend pregnancy state. If it works, the Pill is better than the other drugs for endometriosis because the side effects of those are much more serious, such as a decrease in bone density.

However, the Pill is not as effective for advanced endometriosis and is not suitable for women who want to become pregnant (der). In one study, most women had a return of endo symptoms within six months of stopping the Pill.

The pregnancy rate of women who have endo is also low following the use of the Pill.

Things to take while on the Pill

- The Pill influences a number of nutrients. You'll need more of vitamins B2, B3, B6, folic acid and zinc, but less iron because of the smaller blood loss at the period. If you are on the Pill, a daily B-group vitamin is a good idea, especially one with a B6 level of between 25 and 50 milligrams. (You may be prescribed a larger daily dose.) This may also help with depression and mood changes associated with the Pill.
- Depression can also be tackled by trying a Pill with a lower oestrogen dose.
- Herbal diuretics, especially dandelion leaf tea, can help with fluid retention symptoms. One or two teaspoons a cup, twice daily (not before bed) is the usual dose.

143

Vegetable juices with parsley and celery can also have a diuretic effect, and there are herbal diuretic tablets. Beware of diuretic drugs which can strip the body of potassium. Cut down on salt in food.

- Many women also report that evening primrose oil (between 1 and 3 grams a day) is useful for many of the symptoms, such as fluid retention, that they experience while taking the Pill. Diet can also be altered to take in more essential fatty acids. (See Bad Fats and Good Fats, number 8 of 20 Good-Eating Hints in the Self Care chapter.)

- The blood copper level increases when women are on the Pill and may be partly responsible for the mood changes. High copper levels can lead to a zinc deficiency and zinc supplements may be needed, especially by vegetarians and vegans. A zinc information page is included in the Minerals section of the Self Care chapter. The usual dose of zinc is 15–30 milligrams a day.

- Women who smoke and take the Pill can take 100 IU of vitamin E every day to reduce the risk of blood clot formation (but usually not if you have a pre-existing heart condition or high blood pressure). But quite frankly, you are taking a helluva risk smoking while on the Pill. Even women in their twenties and early thirties can have strokes.

- A balanced diet will help to prevent nutrient deficiencies while on the Pill (for a balanced diet see the 20 Good-Eating Hints in the Self Care chapter).

Things to watch out for while on the Pill

- Blood levels of vitamin A increase while on the Pill, so vitamin A supplements including cod liver oil, should never be taken with the Pill.

  The absorption of betacarotene (the precursor to vitamin A) from food, however, may be lower and so you should eat plenty of orange and yellow vegetables.

- Some drugs can make the Pill a less powerful contraceptive, including some anti-epileptic drugs, some antibiotics and the anti-fungal medication Griseofulvin. Some drugs are cleared more slowly from the body when women are on the Pill. Theophylline, the anti-asthma drug, is one of these.

- Painkillers with paracetamol, like Panadol, reduce the rate at which oestrogen is naturally cleared from the body and may lead to higher levels and more side effects from too much oestrogen.

- Women on thyroid hormones (such as Tertroxine) may need to increase their dose if they are also prescribed the Pill. Some sedatives, tranquillisers and anti-depressant drugs may not work as well; others seem to have a stronger effect, such as the tricyclic anti-depressants Tofranil and Melipramine. If you are on the Pill or prescribed the Pill as well as any other drug, discuss the possible effects with a doctor or at the local chemist.

When to stop the Pill

Symptoms or conditions which indicate that the Pill should be stopped immediately include blood clots, high blood pressure or serious headaches.

Smoking while on the Pill increases the risk of developing those problems.

Post-Pill absence of periods is not usually treated by doctors until you want to get pregnant, when doctors will prescribe fertility drugs like Clomid. (Side effects should be discussed with your doctor.) Until this time, the usual recommendation is for women to go back on the Pill to maintain their bone density because oestrogen levels are lower when you don't ovulate.

Progestogens

The commonly used progesterone-like drugs or 'progestogens' come from two classes—medroxyprogesterone acetate such as Provera, and norethisterone such as Primulut N. Both progestogens are used in the Pill, and are also prescribed for bleeding irregularities, endometriosis and for the menopause. (You may have heard of Depo Provera. This just means an injection of Provera — depo means injected — lasting three months. It is advertised by manufacturers as an easy, long-term contraception. These can be stopped if side effects are a problem. There are other reliable tablet forms of contraception which have fewer side effects.)

Progestogens are often prescribed for heavy periods, even if the patient doesn't have irregularities in progesterone production. When you stop taking the drug, it causes complete shedding of the endometrium, which often stops the abnormal bleeding. These drugs need to be given for about 21 days — usually from Day 5 to Day 25 of the menstrual cycle. They are usually prescribed for between one and three menstrual cycles, but sometimes for longer. The androgen-like side effects and abnormal cholesterol levels associated with Primulut and the norethisterones restrict their use to no more than 6–12 months. They can be prescribed as a component of HRT to menopausal women who are taking oestrogens and who have not had a hysterectomy. The sister book in this series, *Menopause*, has a full run-down on HRT and its risks and benefits.

Provera and Duphaston (dydrogesterone) are the common progestogens used for endometriosis and can either be taken in the last part of the cycle, or taken continuously to create a pregnancy-like state with no period. About 30 per cent of women have spotting and breakthrough bleeding until the drug starts to work or the dose is adjusted. These drugs are relatively inexpensive (compared to some of the others used for endometriosis) and can give significant pain relief to some women without serious long-term side effects.

Possible side effects
Progestogen side effects can include nausea, bloating, acne, breast tenderness, weight gain and mood changes involving a lot of sudden, unexplained shouting (alright, maybe it was just me) which may be related to the blokey hormone effects of the drugs. The medroxyprogesterones such as Provera have fewer blokey hormone effects. Primulut and other norethisterones have mild oestrogenic, anabolic (growth promoting) and blokey hormone effects.

Provera and Duphaston can cause side effects in some women that are a real drag, or should we say drag queen, including increased hairiness, mood changes and a deeper voice. All the symptoms should go away after the drug use stops, except for the deepening of the voice. Singers and actors and people who want to sound like Betty Boop beware: use another drug if you can. Fertility is not improved as a result of using progestogens. The return to a regular cycle may be delayed for many months and there are no studies assessing the return rate of endometriosis after progestogen use.

What to take with progestogens
When side effects from progestogens are a problem, the B vitamins, herbal diuretics or evening primrose oil, and essential fatty acids in the diet can sometimes reduce symptoms. For doses see the recommendations under the Pill, above.

Progesterone
The hormone progesterone (not the progestogens, such as Provera and Primulut) has been used for some time for PMS symptoms. Progesterone cannot be taken in a pill because it is very quickly broken down in the liver. So it has to be taken as either a vaginal pessary, a cream, an injection or a troche (a tablet held in the mouth).

Progesterone has many enthusiastic supporters for its use in treating PMS and breast soreness. This drug is often referred to as 'natural progesterone' because it is made from soy plants or wild yam. Natural or not, however, it is still a drug and should be treated as such. Research on its long-term safety and effectiveness is lacking, so caution is warranted.

Hormone replacement therapy (HRT)

The drugs used for HRT are either oestrogens alone or oestrogens with synthetic progesterone (progestogens). They may come in the form of tablets, patches, or occasionally creams or pessaries. Different types of HRT are used depending on whether you are peri-menopausal or menopausal. Newer hormone-like drugs are Evista and Livial. HRT and these new drugs are explored in detail in the sister book in this series called *Menopause*.

HORMONE-BLOCKING DRUGS

GnRH agonists

We pause for a short message about how the body works. The hypothalamus gland in the brain releases a hormone called gonadotrophin releasing hormone (GnRH). GnRH tells the pituitary gland to start pumping out important hormones which drive the menstrual cycle – luteinising hormone (LH) and follicle stimulating hormone (FSH).

Drugs with a similar chemical structure to GnRH are called GnRH analogues. GnRH analogues either mimic the action or stop you making your own GnRH. When taken continuously, a GnRH analogue stops ovulation and is then called a GnRH agonist – agonist means a competitor. These drugs are mainly used to treat endometriosis and fibroid cysts.

The GnRH agonists are often used to shrink fibroids and the number of blood vessels which surround them before a myomectomy (surgical removal of a fibroid). This is useful simply because it reduces bleeding and

149

makes it easier to remove a smaller fibroid. Another advantage is to reduce heavy periods before the op, which allows you to deal with any anaemia before surgery. Unless surgery follows the use of the GnRH agonists, the fibroid will grow again when you stop taking the drugs.

When taken for endometriosis, the drugs induce a temporary menopausal state. GnRH agonists are equally effective as Danazol in reducing the symptoms and the size of endometrial implants, and the side effects are said to be less severe. Endometrial cysts usually return to their initial size four months after stopping drug treatment, making some sort of additional treatment necessary. GnRH agonists have no extra benefits in improving fertility.

GnRH agonists have also been trialled in combination with the Pill for premenstrual symptoms. These sorts of treatments are controversial because they're pretty heavy drugs, and are reserved for really feral cases of PMS. They are very occasionally used for abnormal bleeding which has failed to respond to other treatment.

GnRH agonists cannot be used as pills because of their chemical make-up. Instead, they are either given as an injection (Zoladex), usually once a month; or as a nostril spray (Synarel). They cause a menopausal state and stop periods during their use. Ovulation usually comes back within about a month of stopping the drugs.

Possible side effects
Menopausal symptoms such as hot flushes, dry vagina and headaches are common, and some women have difficulty with sex because of vaginal dryness. And some women,

come to mention it, find themselves less than interested in the whole idea of sex.

There is an early and significant bone density loss after starting on GnRH agonists. Radial bone density (measured in the wrist) is not affected, but the bone density of the spine shows significant changes. For some women, this may not be reversible and should be considered as part of their decision to use GnRH agonists. Oestrogen and progesterone given together might prevent bone density loss, but aggravate the condition that GnRH agonists were prescribed for.

Some people will develop ovarian cysts in the first two months of treatment with GnRH agonists, especially if they have a previous history of polycystic ovarian syndrome. These cysts will often disappear themselves as the treatment progresses, but can grow large enough to require surgery or going off the drug.

What to take with GnRH agonists

Women who take GnRH agonists should ensure that their calcium and magnesium intake is high enough. Information pages on calcium and magnesium are included in the Minerals section of the Self Care chapter.

Plant oestrogens can help offset menopausal symptoms brought on by using the drugs (more info is under plant oestrogens in the Natural Therapies chapter).

Tamoxifen

Tamoxifen is a synthetic anti-oestrogen drug which is used for women with oestrogen-responsive breast cancer and (controversially) for premenstrual breast pain. Long-term use of this drug is associated with a higher risk of endometrial cancer and uterine polyps. Other side effects include hot flushes; vaginal dryness, itch or discharge; menstrual changes when women are pre-menopausal and bleeding in post-menopausal women.

Prostaglandins-inhibitors

These drugs inhibit the prostaglandins which cause the heavier periods and period pain from increased uterine muscle spasm. They can be bought without a prescription from a chemist. Aspirin is a well-known prostaglandins-inhibitor, but is not much chop for period pain. Some of the newer, more effective ones are Ponstan, Naprogesic, ACT 3 and Nurofen. Prostaglandins-inhibitors are absorbed quickly and can reduce pain in about half an hour. They can be used for the relief of period pain, including the moderate to severe period pain associated with endometriosis. Some women only use them when they have pain, others prefer to start to take them before the expected onset of the period.

There seems to be no difference in effectiveness if the drugs are taken before the start of the period, but it's best to get on to them early if vomiting accompanies pain. Keep the dose in the lowest effective range.

Women who have heavy periods, and who continue to ovulate seem to respond better to these drugs than women who are not ovulating. The drugs also seem to work better in combination with the Pill or progesterone tablets, and some doctors recommend these treatments be combined.

Ponstan has also been used to treat mood swings,

fatigue, headache and the general aches and pains which accompany PMS.

You shouldn't take these drugs for longer than seven days at a time, so they're no good for the many women who experience PMS for more than a week before their period.

Prostaglandins-inhibitors do not actually reverse the prostaglandins imbalance which causes heavy periods, pain or PMS and will have to be used indefinitely until the cause(s) of the imbalance are found and dealt with.

Prostaglandins-inhibitors only control symptoms while they're around. This is not a very alluring prospect, especially since there are many side effects.

Possible side effects
About a quarter of people using prostaglandins-inhibitors have problems with the gastro-intestinal system. Symptoms can include nausea, vomiting, stomach pain, indigestion, diarrhoea, heartburn, abdominal cramps, constipation, abdominal bloating and wind. These drugs should always be taken with food to try to minimise the risk of gastric ulceration. Steer clear of them if you have a history of gastro-intestinal disease.

A number of other complaints can be aggravated by the use of prostaglandins-inhibitors and they may cause problems if you have poor liver function, asthma, clotting disorders, lupus, and heart disease. Prostaglandins-inhibitors can mask the signs of infection and should not be taken when period pain is known or suspected to be caused by pelvic inflammatory disease.

What to take with them

Slippery elm can help to prevent gastric ulceration associated with these drugs. One teaspoon mixed into apple
juice, or into equal quantities of apple juice mixed with
yoghurt, and taken at the same time as the drug, helps to
protect the stomach lining.

DIURETICS

Diuretics have been one of the most commonly prescribed
drugs for bloating and breast tenderness associated with
PMS thought to be caused by fluid retention. The results
of trials using different types of diuretics have been
conflicting, and due to a tendency for some women to
bolt down more tablets than they should, they're not so
often prescribed. Some diuretics deplete potassium, so
check with your doctor about potassium supplements.

ANTI-DEPRESSANTS AND ANXIOLYTICS

A variety of anti-depressants and anxiolytics (anti-anxiety
drugs) are sometimes used for mood disorders associated
with period problems, particularly PMS and around
menopause. As a general rule it's best to stay right away
from them. They treat only the symptoms if they treat
anything at all, and you can become dependent without
getting to the cause of the problem. In some cases the
depression gets more entrenched. The minor tranquillisers, such as the benzodiazepines (Valium) may add to
the fatigue and lethargy often associated with hormonal
changes.

SURGERY

If you've gotta, you've gotta, but don't be afraid of getting a second opinion, or more if you like, before you agree. Except in emergency situations, surgery should be seen as a last resort. Surgery can be necessary for proper diagnosis and/or treatment. In this section we explain the most common gynaecological procedures.

Whatever surgery you're having, make sure you read the hints below about preparing for surgery and better recovery. These days you can be shovelled in and out of hospital so fast, you'll need all the help you can get in recovering. (Don't feel you have to go home the same day, and if you do, make sure somebody can care for you properly. If you're going home alone or to a houseful of screaming kids who need looking after, don't be bullied and insist on the extra day in hospital. The after-effects of general anaesthetic are not to be sneezed at.)

Good pre-operative strategies can make all the difference to recovering quickly and easily from even a major operation.

Anaesthetics

If you're having general anaesthetic you will need to stay in hospital for a minimum of four hours and maybe longer, depending on what procedures you undergo. Anaesthetics are evolving all the time, and have been since they used whisky or a swift blow to the noggin. 'General' anaesthetics will render you unconscious for the duration of the surgery. Different 'generals' are used — anaesthetists often have their own favourites.

Some people react badly to anaesthetics — if you have a second operation after a bad experience recovering from anaesthetic, find out what you had last time and tell the anaesthetist to try something different.

It's increasingly popular to skip the 'pre-med' relaxing shot of pethidine or other drugs, such as Scopolomine, used to dry up secretions. It's now believed that people recover more quickly from anaesthetic after an operation if they don't have a pre-med. Never lie to your anaesthetist about how much you weigh, how much alcohol you drink or how many cigarettes you smoke. This will affect the amount of anaesthetic and drugs you need during surgery.

Hysteroscopy

Reason
To have a look around the inside of the uterus. A diagnostic hysteroscopy is used before any treatment to exclude serious conditions when abnormal bleeding or other worrying symptoms are present, especially when women are over 40. Small procedures such as the removal of polyps or fibroids can be performed at the same time.

Anaesthetic
A general anaesthetic in hospital is recommended by most doctors because, unless you've given birth, your cervix will be too small to pass the instrument through without considerable discomfort. Sometimes a hysteroscopy is performed with a local anaesthetic in the specialist's rooms.

Procedure

A hysteroscope is a small pencil-sized instrument which is inserted into the cervix and through which the inner cavity of the uterus can be seen. The uterine cavity is inflated with gas or fluid so that a good view is possible and extra procedures may be performed. The doctor should be able to see if any parts of the endometrium appear to be diseased.

Time

About half an hour. If a general anaesthetic has been used, there's a four-hour recovery time in hospital. You can probably go home on the same day.

Laparoscopy

Reason

A look around the pelvic organs, usually searching for problems like blocked Fallopian tubes, endometriosis or cysts of some kind. Many kinds of treatment may be performed at the same time, such as removal of cysts, and laser destruction of endometriosis implants.

Anaesthetic

General, in hospital.

Procedure

The surgeon makes two or more small incisions to insert the look-around instrument, called a laparoscope. This thin, pencil-like instrument has fibre-optics through which the operator can view the inner organs. There is usually one incision under the navel and another just above the pubic bone. The abdomen is usually filled with a gas so that it is pumped up with an 'air' making it easier for the surgeon to see each individual organ, and there's more room to move the laparoscope around. At the end of the procedure, most of the gas is forced out, but some stays in the abdominal cavity and can cause pain or discomfort until it eventually dissipates, which can be after a few days. The pressure of the gas affects nerves, and can cause 'referred' pain in the shoulders.

Minor surgical procedures can be performed during a laparoscopy, such as removing patches of endometriosis with laser (which vaporises) or diathermy (burning off with electrical current), the removal of small ovarian cysts, and the removal of adhesions. These procedures usually only involve a day in hospital; and pain and post-operative complications are minimal because the incisions are small.

Time

Sometimes you can go home the same day, sometimes the next day, depending on what had to be done. A quick look around is one thing, but additional surgery like laser treatment will add on to your recovery time.

Recovery time is usually a few days depending on the extent of the additional surgery and the type of complaint treated. Even though the external wounds can be quite small, the internal organs might take a while to recover. Pain is a good indicator of how much to do and when rest is needed. Listen to your body. See the advice below on pre- and post-op care: it's important.

Laparotomy

Reason
For more extensive surgery than a laparoscopy can handle. Often, to remove large cysts, endometriosis, or to do some repair work to help with fertility.

Anaesthetic
General, in hospital.

Procedure
A laparotomy involves an abdominal incision, usually just above the pubic bone and can include removal of extensive and hard-to-reach adhesions, removal of larger ovarian cysts, diathermy (burning off with electrical current) or laser (vaporising) of extensive and difficult-to-reach endometriosis, or for reconstruction and microsurgery of reproductive bits. For example, a laparotomy is usual when emergency surgery has to be performed for a ruptured ectopic pregnancy.

Time
A laparotomy can take from between half an hour and several hours, depending on the type of surgery to be performed. Recovery time is longer than after a laparoscopy because the abdominal wounds are more extensive and so is the internal surgery. You may be in hospital a few days to a week.

Endometrial ablation

Reason
Usually to counter heavy periods. The preferred outcome is that only a little or no endometrium is left behind.

There are many critics of this procedure, and disadvantages include a high failure rate. Periods often continue, especially when the patient has adenomyosis. For some though, when all other treatments have failed, this procedure offers a possible alternative to the conventional hysterectomy.

Anaesthetic
General, in hospital.

Procedure
An endometrial ablation is destruction of the lining of the uterus (endometrium) either with a laser or by cauterisation. A hysteroscope (see above) is inserted through the vagina and cervix and into the uterus to perform the operation.

Time
Usually half an hour to three-quarters of an hour.

'D&C' (dilatation and curettage) or curette/termination

Reason
Usually performed after a miscarriage to make sure all tissue is removed, and to reduce the risk of haemorrhage. It is also the surgical procedure used for pregnancy termi-

nation. (There is a way of causing an early termination by the use of a hormonal drug, but that drug has been effectively disallowed in Australia by the Federal Government, meaning women who need a termination are denied a choice between surgery and a tablet.) Curettes are also used to remove the endometrium to test it for cancerous or pre-cancerous cells in a laboratory. A D&C can also be performed for diagnostic reasons.

Anaesthetic
General, in hospital. Some doctors will use a local anaesthetic injection to the cervix.

Procedure
The surface of the endometrial lining of the uterus is scraped away with a surgical instrument. The surface begins to grow back straight away and is back to normal within a few weeks.

Time
Usually about ten minutes.

Myomectomy

Reason
To surgically remove one or more fibroids without removing the uterus. This can be a difficult operation to perform. Some points for and against myomectomy and hysterectomy are discussed below.

Usually a gynaecologist will recommend that a fibroid be removed in these cases:

- fibroids larger than a 12–14 week pregnancy
- fibroids that are growing
- fibroids associated with heavy bleeding
- the fibroid is pedunculated (attached to a stem)
- the fibroid interferes with fertility

Surgery or not?

Size is often quoted as a reason for removing a fibroid, whether it is causing symptoms or not. In direct opposition to this recommendation, a recent comment in the *American Journal of Obstetrics and Gynecology* suggested that regardless of size, the presence and severity of significant symptoms 'should be the most important considerations in the individualization of treatment strategies'. In other words, if it's not causing problems, leave it alone.

Fibroids are also blamed for problems with fertility and removal is sometimes suggested before you try to get pregnant, just in case. It is unlikely, however, that the fibroids will affect fertility and conception rates. The same study showed that there was an increased rate of caesarean section when a woman has fibroids, particularly if they are situated in the lower portion of the uterus, but no change in fertility rate. Women with fibroids have an increased risk of severe bleeding following childbirth caused by the fibroid interfering with uterine contractions.

Myomectomy or hysterectomy?

For women past their childbearing years or those who don't want to get pregnant, a hysterectomy is usually recommended. For others, a myomectomy may be suggested.

Some surgeons are reluctant to perform a myomectomy, especially for women who don't want to have (more) children. It's difficult for even the most experienced surgeon to predict how easily a fibroid can be removed. You could bleed severely, and this may mean that a hysterectomy will have to be performed anyway, and under less than optimum conditions. Sometimes the exact location of the fibroid will only be discovered during the surgery.

It may be in a position where it is difficult to reach, or surrounded by delicate structures. It may be fed by more blood vessels than usual.

Other reasons for not wanting to perform a myomectomy are that the fibroids may grow back or the heavy period bleeding associated with the fibroid prior to its removal may not stop. An unspoken reason for suggesting hysterectomy is the common medical opinion that women who do not intend to have a child have no need for a uterus. A hysterectomy may be offered first and a myomectomy discussed only if you mention it.

This decision is often difficult for many women. When a hysterectomy has been advised, but is not a suitable option, a second opinion from a gynaecologist experienced in the technique of myomectomy is advisable.

Removal of fibroids using laser is reported to reduce bleeding at the time of surgery, reduce the risk of adhesions and improve the fertility rate of women wanting to conceive.

Sometimes a hysterectomy may be the only option. A myomectomy might just be too risky, complicated or unpredictable. There may be too many fibroids (although we know of a 45-year-old whose gynaecologist removed 42 fibroids rather than perform a hysterectomy!) or there may be other gynaecological reasons why a hysterectomy is a better option.

Both hysterectomy and myomectomy are elective procedures and so it is possible to arrange an auto-transfusion (where a woman gives her own blood some days before the operation and then is transfused with this blood during the procedure if needed). If you give blood for an auto-transfusion, take iron supplements and increase your daily intake of iron-containing foods (see the info page on iron in the Minerals sections of the Self Care chapter).

Anaesthetic
General, in hospital.

Procedure
It is usually performed through a laparotomy incision. The fibroids are cut out with a scalpel and care must be taken to stop all the bleeding.

Time
The procedure usually takes up to two hours.

Hysterectomy

Reason

This procedure is a last resort in several conditions including really severe, unresponsive endometriosis, heavy periods, fibroids, the severe pain and bleeding associated with adenomyosis and other serious gynaecological conditions, and some cancers. Sometimes doctors talk about a 'partial hysterectomy' (removal of the uterus but not the ovaries).

Anaesthetic

General, in hospital.

Procedure

A hysterectomy is the removal of the uterus, but the removal of the uterus and Fallopian tubes and ovaries is generally also known as a hysterectomy. Its technical term is bilateral salpingo-oophorectomy. (Sometimes you really do have to worry about doctors. Oophorectomy indeed.) A 'total hysterectomy' usually means that the cervix is taken as well as the uterus, and a 'sub-total' hysterectomy usually means the cervix is left alone. Make sure you understand exactly what your doctor means when the word hysterectomy is used. The operation can be done by making an incision in the stomach and cutting out the uterus; or by entering the body through the vagina with surgical instruments, cutting away the uterus, and pulling it out through the vagina. (Sorry to get a bit graphic, but that's what happens.)

A hysterectomy for endometriosis will probably be done through an abdominal incision if there are multiple adhesions which make vaginal removal too difficult. For conditions which are oestrogen-dependent, such as severe and non-responsive endometriosis and some types of cancer, the removal of the uterus and ovaries is often recommended. Removing the ovaries can prevent or slow growth of these oestrogen-responsive tissues but, of course, means you will become menopausal.

Time
This is a major operation. It usually takes three-quarters of an hour to an hour, but can take several hours depending on possible complications. You will probably be in hospital for between five and ten days.

PREPARING FOR SURGERY

The following pre-surgery hints will help you to improve wound healing and reduce wound infections; assist with getting up and around again as quickly as possible; and cut down on the common discomfort of bowel problems after surgery, caused by your inside bits being disturbed.

The hints will help in any abdominal surgery, including hysterectomy, myomectomy, laparoscopy, laser surgery, laparotomy or caesarean section. Check them with your surgeon.

- Give up smoking — for good if you can, but at least for two weeks before the operation. This will reduce your risk of post-operative chest infections.

- A few dietary changes in the week before surgery can help to prevent or reduce the symptoms of bowel problems afterwards.
- Eat daily salads of grated raw carrot and beetroot or a medium-sized cooked beetroot.
- Yoghurt or cultured milk drinks colonise the bowel with healthy bacteria and cut down on painful wind. Drink or eat about one cup a day of yoghurt with live cultures and no sugar. (Jalna, Hakea and Gippsland are good brands with low-fat options.)
- Avoid refined sugars which tend to increase bowel fermentation and wind.
- Avoid foods which usually cause you wind, constipation or diarrhoea.
- If you already have irritable bowel syndrome or suffer from sensitive bowels: in the week before the op, have three to six cups daily of a special herbal tea combination. Make up a jar with equal parts of *Melissa officinalis* (lemon balm), *Matricaria recutita* (chamomile) and *Mentha piperita* (peppermint tea). Use 2 teaspoons of the mixture for each cup of tea. Take it with you to hospital, and continue taking it for the week after the operation.
- Post-operative nausea is relieved by common ginger root. The usual dose is between $1/2$ and 1 gram every four hours, in tablet form, or between 10 and 20 drops as a fluid oral extract. Organise to take this to the hospital with you to start using as soon as you can after the surgery, but check with the medical staff first.
- Get your muscles going. Poor muscle strength and agility can slow down recovery because getting out of

bed and walking around is much more difficult. Weak leg and abdominal muscles can be improved by specific exercises such as yoga exercises, squats, walking, sit-ups and gym work. About a month is usually needed to dramatically improve muscle strength but even a few days before the op is better than nothing.

- Vitamin C has been shown to improve wound healing time. Start at least one week before surgery on about 2 grams a day and keep going for three to four weeks afterwards.

- Make sure you're getting enough zinc. A lot of women don't. Zinc supplements also have a beneficial effect on wound healing, but probably only in zinc-deficient people. Start a good zinc supplement, such as around 75–150 milligrams of zinc chelate a day with food for two or three weeks before the operation and continue for about two weeks afterwards. (There's an info page about zinc under Minerals in the Self Care chapter.)

- Vitamin E, which prevents internal scar tissue formation (adhesions), is great when fertility must be conserved following surgery. Doses of around 100–250 IU should be taken two weeks before the surgery but stopped two days before the operation. This is a relatively small dose, because of a very slight risk of increased bleeding during surgery. Once you can eat again after the operation you can take doses of around 400 or 500 IU a day until you're recovered. This will reduce the risk of post-operative blood clots. Vitamin E cream can also be rubbed into the wound to speed up healing and reduce scarring.

RECOVERING FROM SURGERY

People have forgotten how to convalesce. With the increase in laser surgery, and the resulting shorter hospital stays, some patients are sent home the day after surgery or even the day of the operation.

Many women start housework, child care or go back to work within days of surgical procedures and then wonder why they spend the rest of the year feeling so awful. The financial strains on the average household also mean that many people feel they 'can't afford' to convalesce properly.

Don't take too much notice of standard doctors' predictions of 'you'll be back at the gym in a week' or 'you'll be up and walking by tomorrow'. Everybody is different. Our completely unscientific, informal survey of women who have had abdominal surgery revealed that almost all of them took longer to recover than their doctors suggested they would, and felt there was something wrong with their constitution, not with what the doctor told them.

Any surgery can take longer than expected, with much intrusive moving around of your inside bits. The standard recovery prediction then becomes even less relevant to you, but sometimes you won't be given a re-assessment of your convalescent time.

Recovery times vary considerably between individuals and are influenced by factors such as smoking, lack of previous fitness, an inability to take it easy and let the body heal, having to get up and look after the kids or go back to work before you're ready, as well as more surgery than was originally planned.

It's better to be guided by pain and stamina and to do a little more every day than to resume former levels of work and exercise too quickly. In other words: go by how you feel, not by a standard information sheet given out by the hospital, which will often be based only on averages or best-case scenarios and written by somebody with no first-hand experience.

When the body is under stress or recovering from an illness, it needs heaps more nutrients than usual. Unfortunately, this often happens just when you've lost your appetite. (Any stress, whether it be from surgery, difficult times, a car accident, or too much work, has a similar effect on the body's need for nutrients.) Being physically active after the procedure improves recovery time and stamina, and reduces the risk of blood clots and respiratory infections. This does not mean you can start doing aerobics the day after. It means you start shuffling around in your slippers as soon as you can and build up from there.

- Your recovering body needs a boost of protein, the B vitamins — particularly vitamin B5 (pantothenic acid), vitamin C, potassium, magnesium and zinc. You can have a daily vitamin B complex tablet which has 50 milligrams of B5 and B6, with a multi-mineral supplement and 1–2 grams of powdered vitamin C until you feel on top of things again.
- To keep energy steady, eat small but frequent meals of complex carbohydrate (potato, rice, bread, oatmeal and pasta), combined with small amounts of protein

such as yoghurt, cheese, tofu, hommos, tuna or egg until your normal appetite and bowel function comes back.

- Avoid any food which acts as a 'body stressor', such as caffeine, refined sugars and huge strawberry daiquiris, until you've recovered.
- Some exercise is vital. Exercise every second day allows for one day of recovery after energy expenditure. As strength improves, exercise every day will increase stamina and a sense of wellbeing. Exercise should be taken at a much slower pace. People tend to overestimate their capabilities so a good rule of thumb is to start at half the level you imagine you could comfortably manage now; if it is too little, no harm will be done. Long slow distance exercise is best — especially walking.
- Simple, easily digested soups and 'energy drinks' provide concentrated nutrients.
- Have one serve of a cooked green leafy vegetable such as spinach, Chinese cabbage or silverbeet every day during the recovery period.
- Never skip breakfast and have a cooked breakfast (porridge, egg on toast, cooked rice cereal, vegetable soup) at least every second day.
- Use the suggested menus given for the hypoglycaemic diet coming up on pages 185–8.

Soups are useful recovery foods. The best types are ones based on grains, especially barley and rice; legumes, such as tofu, orange lentils, fresh soya beans and red kidney

171

beans (but not if they give you wind); or root vegies like potato, carrot and sweet potato.

Chicken broth
Yes, the old stand-by, traditional comfort food. Use free-range chicken carcasses. The broth can be prepared with a particular flavour. For example, Thai (lemongrass, lime leaves, galangal, and chilli), or Western (celery, bay leaves, onion, carrot and peppercorns).

High-protein drinks
High-protein drinks are useful meal substitutes or for between meals, particularly if you don't feel hungry and you're having trouble digesting.

ALMOND SMOOTHIE
2 dessertspoons almond meal
1 teaspoon rice bran
1 teaspoon wheatgerm

Blend with:
1 cup commercial soya milk (Bonsoy, Aussie Soy, Vitasoy) and
   1 teaspoon malt extract
or
1/2 cup yoghurt and 1/2 cup fruit juice

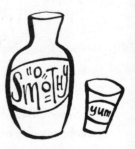

BERRY DRINK

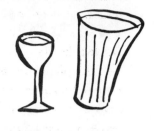

1/2 punnet blueberries, strawberries,
    raspberries or other berry fruit
    in season
1/2–3/4 cup yoghurt or soya milk
    (yoghurt and berries tend to be
    fairly tangy and may not be to
    everyone's liking)
1 dessertspoon almond meal, ground cashews, or seeds

Blend together until smooth.

TOFU DRINKS
50 grams soft tofu

Blend with any of the following combinations:

6 dried apricots (soaked overnight in a cup of water) and
    the water they have been soaked in
2 dessertspoons almond meal
1 teaspoon slippery elm powder
or
1 banana
1 teaspoon slippery elm powder *or* 1 teaspoon rice bran
1 dessertspoon almond meal
1 cup fruit juice
or
1 glass freshly squeezed orange juice
1–2 dessertspoons almond meal *or* ground cashew nuts
1 teaspoon slippery elm powder

Natural Therapies

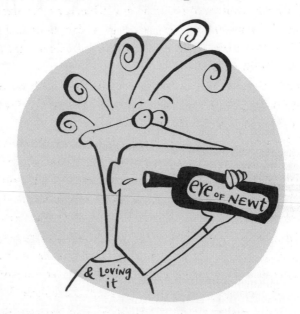

CHOOSING AND WORKING WITH YOUR NATURAL THERAPIST

Natural therapists to avoid are ones who have to work sitting under a pyramid for the 'vibes'; ones who insist that they are 'healers' (Blue heelers, maybe); ones who explain that most of their knowledge is based on 'intuitive' messages from the Great Beyond; and ones who say there is no value, under any circumstances, in scientific medicine. Here are some hints on how to narrow the field:

- Familiarise yourself with the different disciplines of natural therapy explained in this section, and decide which kind of practitioner might suit you best.
- Find out what professional qualifications the therapist has, how recent their training is and how they keep abreast, and what professional organisations your therapist belongs to.
- Many natural therapists prescribe herbs. It is best if herbs are prescribed by a full member of the National Herbalists' Association of Australia.
- Your practitioner should, at least, be affiliated with the major governing group for their discipline. (The National Herbalists' Association of Australia requires 700 hours of relevant study for membership; equivalent State bodies also require 700 hours, the Australian Natural Therapists' Association requires 700 hours study in an approved course; and the Australian Traditional Medicine Society requires no specific number of hours for each discipline.)
- Regardless of their qualifications, you have to like and trust your therapist. Don't be afraid to shop around.
- Try to find a natural therapist who specialises in your problem.
- Any treatment must target the underlying cause, not just the symptoms: you need a full diagnosis as well as treatment. For example, if you have heavy bleeding, don't accept a preparation to stop it without knowing the gynaecological cause. If you simply mask important symptoms, you might be hiding an underlying problem that your body is trying to warn you about.

This means you may have to have medical tests then return to the natural therapist armed with the results.

- Some crucial examinations are not performed by natural therapists and referral to a doctor is needed. The results of the tests can be used by a natural therapist, or a doctor, or both, as a base for their diagnosis and treatment. These include routine screens like Pap tests and breast exams; gynaecological examinations which are performed vaginally and involve internal 'examination' of the pelvic organs; pathology tests such as blood tests, swabs or urine tests; radiological examinations such as ultrasounds and X-rays; and diagnostic operations such as a laparoscopy, a procedure used to look around the pelvic organs, usually searching for problems like blocked Fallopian tubes, endometriosis or cysts of some kind.

- Be suspicious of practitioners who prescribe vast amounts of herbs or supplements from their clinic at inflated prices. Four different preparations is a fairly average prescription. If you go home with a plastic bag with 15 different pills, powders and potions, a bunch of pussy willows and seven sacks of dandelion tea, you should be asking why you need it all. It is quite proper for a natural therapist to dispense from their own clinic, just make sure that if they sell you over-the-counter products, for example, Blackmore's, that their price is competitive with say, your local supermarket. This goes for health food shops too.

- Be wary of any doctor or natural therapist who has a hard and fast pet theory which they apply to all situations — examples of these are people who claim that most disorders, from period pain to exhaustion are caused only by the liver, or stress, or dehydration, or toxicity, or the fact that the moon in June was in Pisces.

- Always tell the natural therapist anything you think is relevant to your condition. This definitely includes other medications you're on, including drugs, herbs or supplements (including vitamins).
- Always follow the instructions on herbal prescriptions and supplements exactly. Never assume that just because something is 'natural' you can take as much as you want to, or vary the recommended doses. Like drugs, under some circumstances, herbs can be dangerous.
- If you are not happy with the results of treatment, seek a second or further opinion.
- Don't expect a natural therapist to be able to 'cure' everything. There are some conditions which are not satisfactorily treated by natural methods.

THE HOLISTIC PHILOSOPHY

All areas of medicine, including science, have become more interested in the holistic philosophy with its emphasis on the body and mind and a belief in the body wanting to heal itself.

The holistic approach is all about treating individuals with conditions and not just about treating diseases. But it is more than that. It is also about listening to a person's own take on their health. For example, let's say you have a lower pelvic pain. You're poked and prodded and questioned and every avenue is pursued. Your doctor says there is nothing wrong. But you're still in pain. Whaddayer mean there's nothing wrong? From a holistic perspective there may be no disease, but something is wrong — your pain indicates some form of disharmony.

This demonstrates another of the important differences between the old and new styles of health care. Medicine usually sees health as an absence of a disease, and illness as an observable or diagnosed disease. Holism sees health as a sense of positive wellness combined with the absence of disease. It makes a further distinction between being ill and having a disease.

A disease is a condition which can be defined by a technique such as blood tests or X-rays. Illness is a perceived sense of feeling sick or being unwell which may or may not be related to a disease. Functional disorders fall into this category. The organs may not be functioning correctly, but there are no signs of changes at a cellular level and routine tests remain within the normal range.

A muscle cramp is a good example of a functional disorder. The muscle is not diseased, even though there is excruciating pain. The muscle is behaving abnormally. The abnormal behaviour could be caused by many different things, and it might be a temporary pain which will never happen again. But the cramp is real and the body is indicating the presence of some sort of disharmony.

Many gynaecological conditions are classed as functional disorders, including most types of period pain and many conditions caused by hormone imbalance such as PMS. Many of the syndromes described by natural therapists are also functional disorders, for example, functional hypoglycaemia and adrenal exhaustion. It's impossible to diagnose these conditions with blood tests, but their response to traditional treatments is reproducible and predictable.

THE TRADITIONS OF NATURAL THERAPY

Today, a good natural therapist will acknowledge the advances in scientific medicine, but base their knowledge on many of the earlier traditions of medicine, including Asian and European herbal and diagnostic methods. Throughout the history of medicine a number of cultures have described remarkably similar systems for recognising health and disease. These include Greek, Roman, Arabic, Indian, Tibetan and Chinese territories. If you didn't know better you'd think all the ancient herbalists from different continents used to have mobile phone conferences and pinch each other's ideas.

The recurring themes had four major aspects: the belief in a 'vital force' as the living and generative energy in the body; the understanding that the universe is composed of a number of 'elements' which are found in varying concentrations in all life forms; the recognition of the potentially damaging influence of extreme weather changes; and the designation of 'constitutional' types to individuals in order to define a predictable framework for diagnosis and treatment.

Throughout the world, climate was respected as a health issue. Normal exposure generated life, but extremes caused death, disease, or at the very least, disruption in the supply of food. And in the case of, say floods, extreme grumpiness. Exposure to wind, cold, dry, damp or heat as a cause of disease was a handy explanation because the weather affected everybody and was easily understood.

Eventually, a classification of diseases according to 'quality' was adopted throughout much of the world. Any complaint accompanied by heat, fever, redness or itchiness, for example, was a Hot condition. Combinations of qualities were also found in each of the elements. Air, for example, was Hot and Moist; Fire was Hot and Dry.

Scientific medicine concerns itself with cellular changes, biochemical phenomena and dissection of the body into its parts. It developed the approach that, for example, the root of one medical problem was a diseased liver. The natural therapies approach is that an underlying disharmony in the whole body was causing the liver disease. In traditional philosophies, it is the lack of harmony and not the disease that is the starting point for treatment.

A good natural therapist will chuck out the information from the past that's no longer useful, and retain the stuff that is still working, for example, a tried and tested herbal remedy.

In the same way, scientific medicine has discarded one theory of the Middle Ages — that the womb wandered around the body — and recently revived another, the use of leeches to deal with certain bruising and strokes.

TYPES OF NATURAL THERAPY

Natural medicine is a generic term which covers any of the therapeutic disciplines that do not use drugs or invasive techniques (like surgery and tests). In Australia, the common practitioners are: naturopaths, herbalists, homoeopaths, acupuncturists, practitioners of traditional Chinese medicine (TCM), aromatherapists, all of the masseurs using various techniques, osteopaths and chiropractors.

Practitioners who use natural therapies may specialise or they may train in a variety of disciplines. A practitioner who uses the multidisciplinary approach has usually trained as a naturopath. Naturopathy is not made up of a specified group of disciplines and each of the colleges may train their students differently. If you're going to a naturopath, ask what disciplines they use before you make the appointment.

The quality of training is extremely varied and there are no regulations in Australia governing the practice of natural therapies. (A butcher could prescribe herbs and be within the law.) Many practitioners are not happy about this and most belong to professional associations as a way of ensuring their educational standing and to demonstrate their commitment to improving the status of their profession.

Here are the most popular disciplines:

Naturopathy The use of any or all of the techniques listed below, usually with a holistic philosophy.

Herbal medicine The prescription of herbs for the treatment of complaints. Prescriptions are usually based on the philosophical doctrine of medical herbalism, not as a straight substitute for drugs.

Homoeopathy Based on the law of the minimum dose and 'like cures like', homoeopathy is the treatment of disease by minute doses of remedies that in healthy persons would produce symptoms like those of the disease.

Acupuncture The insertion of specialised acupuncture needles to regulate and stimulate the body's energy flow, known as Qi (pronounced Chee).

Traditional Chinese medicine (TCM) The use of acupuncture, herbs, and the manipulation of the flow of Qi with massage and specific exercises.

Aromatherapy The use of 'essential oils' as therapeutic agents. They are usually burned in an oil burner to scent the atmosphere or applied to the skin, appropriately diluted in oil, usually about 5 drops to 100 millilitres to be safe.

Massage Massages may be relaxing or 'therapeutic'. A therapeutic massage involves deep tissue massage for the relief of injury, muscular spasm and tension. A relaxation massage is usually more gentle and is designed to relieve stress.

Chiropractic and osteopathy The mobilisation and manipulation of the skeletal structures along with the strengthening and stretching of the muscular components of the body.

Not every natural therapist will adopt a holistic approach, nor will they always involve their clients in the decisions about treatments. A constant belief should be that the restoration of health is more important than treating a particular disease.

BLOOD SUGAR ABNORMALITIES – FUNCTIONAL HYPOGLYCAEMIA

It may be necessary for you to adapt your diet, take supplements or herbs if your practitioner suspects functional hypoglycaemia. Functional hypoglycaemia occurs when there are fluctuations in the blood sugar levels.

Causes

In the normal course of events, you eat a well-balanced meal which causes your blood sugar levels to become pleasantly elevated. Then there is a gently undulating decline of the blood sugar levels until the next well-balanced meal, so the levels remain pretty stable.

Functional hypoglycaemia can be brought on by many things such as prolonged periods of stress, a number of dietary factors affecting blood sugar levels including too much refined carbohydrates and sugars, hitting the grog without eating at the same time, or drinking alcohol with sugar-based mixers. In other words, a glass of wine at dinner is probably fine, but go easier on ordering the Fluffy Poindexter Cointreau and cream pineapple daiquiri rocket fuel cocktail in a coconut shell with three paper umbrellas. Especially if you want to eat the paper umbrellas.

People who go on short-term diets often get hypoglycaemic because their diets are badly designed and don't provide enough energy. Starving, they 'break out' and eat large amounts of starchy or sugary foods. The rapid drop in blood sugar starts a pattern of sugar craving, hypoglycaemic symptoms, and weight gain. The hypoglycaemic

183

diet is a successful way to lose weight slowly and progressively because it breaks the cycle of 'fast and feast'.

Hypoglycaemia just means low blood sugar levels. Functional hypoglycaemia means that this is a disorder of function rather than the blood sugar fluctuations seen with diabetes when there is an actual problem with production of insulin in the pancreas.

If you have PMS or are excessively stressed, following the hypoglycaemic diet usually helps; and if you have PCOS or are very overweight, additional attention to the types of foods to control insulin resistance will also be useful. More of that later in this section.

Symptoms of functional hypoglycaemia

- Tiredness, vagueness or shakiness which goes away when you eat.
- Tiredness or irritability first thing in the morning or if meals are late.
- Sugar cravings.
- Being hungry all the time or soon after eating.
- Headaches when meals are delayed.
- Inappropriate feelings of anxiety or inadequacy which disappear after eating.
- Waking up in the night feeling really hungry.

General dietary guidelines for functional hypoglycaemia

- Eat small amounts of protein regularly at meals and with snacks.
- Eat small meals often — three small meals with three small between-meal snacks.

- Eat wholegrain foods; avoid white flour and refined cereals.
- Avoid all sugar, honey and dried fruit.
- Consume only small quantities of unsweetened, diluted fruit juice.
- Avoid all stimulants such as tea, coffee, chocolate, and cola drinks.
- Avoid alcohol and cigarettes.
- Always eat breakfast.

Protein

All animal protein is 'complete', and therefore meals containing milk products, eggs, meat or fish provide first class protein. Incomplete (plant) protein foods, however, need to be combined with complementary foods and eaten at the same meal to provide the same quality protein as animal protein.

Eat beans with grains: tofu (from soya beans) and rice; lentils and rice; corn and beans; buckwheat and tempeh; muesli and soya milk; kidney beans and barley.

Or eat beans with seeds: tahini and beans; tofu and sesame seeds.

Or eat grains with nuts, nut butters on bread; rice and cashews; rice and peanut sauce.

Morning kick-start

Start the day with one of these:
- the juice of a lemon diluted in a glass of warm water
- half a grapefruit
- citrus juice
- a whole piece of fruit

(We're not suggesting that's your whole breakfast, but have one of them before anything else. It will wake up your digestive process.)

Breakfast ideas

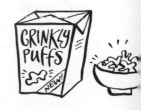

- Home-made muesli: raw oatmeal, rice flakes, puffed millet, sunflower seeds, linseeds, chopped almonds or cashews, coconut and chopped pumpkin seeds. Add low-fat cow's milk, yoghurt or soya milk, and chopped fresh fruit.
- Fresh fruit in season with yoghurt and seeds or chopped nuts.
- Wholegrain bread, toasted with poached egg, nut butter, hommos, low-fat cheese, miso, alfalfa or other sprouts. You don't need butter with these spreads. Avoid honey and jams.
- Cooked cereal such as oatmeal, millet meal, brown rice or buckwheat, with added seeds or soya grits. Add milk of choice and cook with fresh fruit such as pear, peach or apple.
- Energy drink: blend together low-fat yoghurt with either fresh fruit of your choice such as berries, peach, pear or mango (about half and half), and add a teaspoon each of rice bran, ground linseeds, almond meal, wheatgerm, and sunflower seeds.

Lunch ideas

- Wholegrain bread sandwich with a mixture of salad vegies. Include protein such as tuna, salmon, egg, low-fat cheese, marinated tofu, or hommos.

- A salad of mixed vegies such as lettuce salad, coleslaw, tabouli salad, grated beetroot, tomatoes, carrot or celery. Protein should be included either in the form of correctly combined vegetable proteins or animal proteins as above.
- Soup with the addition of beans and grains, yoghurt or parmesan cheese.
- Any of the dinner choices or the breakfast energy drink.

Dinner ideas

Dinner should contain at least five different vegies, cooked or raw depending on season and preference; some protein; and a serve of complex carbohydrate like rice, root vegies, beans, or pasta.

To keep animal protein to a minimum, combine meat with grain or bean dishes. Examples might be lamb and chickpea casserole, or a similar combination, common in the Middle East and the south eastern European countries; pasta and tomato sauce with tuna; stir-fry vegetables with a little meat, and served with rice, common in Asia. Or:

- Steamed vegetables with rice and tofu.
- Stir-fry beef and vegetables with rice.
- Steamed vegetables with lentils and rice.
- Grilled or baked fish with vegetables or salad.
- Minestrone soup with beans and parmesan cheese.

Morning, afternoon or supper snacks

Choose from:
- A small handful of mixed seeds and nuts.

- Half a banana with seeds and nuts.
- A glass of soya milk with pumpkin seeds.
- A small container of low-fat yoghurt.
- Two wholegrain dry biscuits with nut butters, sardines, tuna or hommos.
- Energy drink: Blend together half a cup of fresh fruit or juice, half a cup of low-fat yoghurt, and seeds with a small handful of almonds, and/or wheatgerm and lecithin.
- A small amount of avocado and tuna dressed with balsamic vinegar.

Fluids

- Limit caffeine-containing beverages to two cups of coffee or four cups of tea (and you know that doesn't mean you can have two megajolt triple caffeine-screaming long blacks).
- Drink at least 2 litres of water daily.

Supplements

Magnesium

200–800 milligrams daily of elemental magnesium in the form of magnesium phosphate, aspartate, orotate or chelate.

Zinc

Usual recommended daily allowance is 15–20 mg, but doses up of to 25–50 mg of elemental zinc may be needed to assist with blood sugar abnormalities. Usual sources are as an amino acid chelate of gluconate.

Manganese

Levels of 10mg per day in foods are the usual recommendation for maintaining health. When blood sugar abnormalities occur, supplements containing up to 10mg of manganese may be recommended twice daily.

Chromium

Chromium requirements are higher in those who eat vast amounts of sugar in the diet. The usual daily recommendation is 50 micrograms, but supplements of 200 micrograms daily may be prescribed.

Herbs

Herbs that can help with blood sugar fluctuations include *Gymnema sylvestra* (gymnema), *Galagea officinalis* (goat's rue), *Trigonella foenum-graecum* (fenugreek).

The bitters have a stabilising effect on blood sugar by regulating the secretion of insulin by the pancreas.

BLOOD SUGAR ABNORMALITIES – INSULIN RESISTANCE

Insulin is the hormone responsible for transporting energy-giving glucose into the cells in the body. When insulin resistance occurs, the cells are starved of their energy source, but the levels of insulin in the blood are elevated. This gives rise to higher blood fat levels and causes more fat to be stored leading to weight gain. Not only that, the starved cells give the body the message that more food is needed to solve the problem and the usual result is increased sugar cravings. To top it all off, the muscle bulk declines and fatigue is a common everyday event. The causes of this phenomenon are many, but eating a diet of refined carbohydrates, not exercising regularly (exercise helps glucose enter cells) and deficiencies of nutrients such as chromium, manganese and zinc are all implicated. Women with PCOS seem to inherit a tendency to insulin resistance and many need to follow the diet outlined below to help control their symptoms.

General dietary guidelines for insulin resistance

- Eat carbohydrate foods that have not been refined, such as grains and legumes that have an intact fibrous outer coat. This slows down the speed at which food is digested and allows for a slower release of sugars into the bloodstream, giving more energy over a longer period and reducing the appetite.
- Carbohydrate foods with a low glycaemic index (low GI foods) such as dense breads, long grain Basmati and Doongara rice, sweet or new potatoes (rather than ordinary potato), pasta, noodles, legumes, oat meal and muesli, temperate climate fruit like apples, pears, citrus and stone fruits are more slowly broken down and absorbed, helping to control insulin levels.
- Three small meals with three small between-meal snacks seems to improve impaired glucose tolerance and assist with weight loss. This regime is described in the hypoglycaemic diet section above.
- Restrict the volume of carbohydrate eaten at each main

meal (even if it's the low GI type) to the amount that is equivalent to the size of the palm of your hand. Pasta meals are often much larger than this and will need to be limited if they make up the majority of your meals.

- Losing weight generally will help with insulin resistance, so try also:
- Cutting fats down, but beware of cutting out the good fats (see the section on Bad Fats and Good Fats in the Self Care chapter).
- A dessertspoon of vinegar or lemon juice eaten with a meal (as a dressing for example) slows down stomach emptying, lowers blood sugar and gives the sensation of being fuller for longer.
- Some additional reading on this subject can be found in *The Glucose Revolution: G.I. Plus*, by Jennie Brand-Miller and Kaye Foster-Powell.

THE LIVER

To say that natural therapists are into the liver is an understatement. It has always been considered important. These days, it has become such a scapegoat that while doctors vaguely say 'it's your hormones, dear', some natural therapists blame everything on the liver, and some people think a diet which 'cleanses' the liver will fix everything. Balderdash, poppycock, and furthermore, pish-tosh.

It is, however, the focus of heaps and heaps of disorders and illnesses investigated by natural therapists, and a healthy, working liver is known to be a great advantage for all women.

Back in the Middle Ages, the humoural theory described two personality types or temperaments related to bile and the liver — the choleric and the melancholic. The choleric person was hot-tempered and irascible. Even now, this filters through when we still describe a bad-tempered person as 'liverish'.

The symptoms of liver disharmony described by traditional Chinese medicine include irritability, depression, frustration, anger, and digestive upsets, and common gynaecological complaints such as PMS, irregular periods, light periods or no periods, infertility and period pain.

Many of the broader concepts of the humoural theory and liver dysfunction are incorporated into the herbalist's diagnosis and treatment today. Herbs and foods which improve liver function are used to treat conditions accompanied by emotional symptoms, such as PMS; and conditions caused by hormonal imbalance such as fibrocystic breast disease, endometriosis, fibroids, and some types of excessive bleeding.

Liver function is adversely affected by poor diet; overeating; excessive intake of fats, sugars, alcohol, and coffee; and the ever-increasing burden of environmental poisons.

As the major organ of detoxification in the body, the liver must be ready to process about 3000 chemicals which can be added to foods during processing, and another 12 000 or so chemicals which can be used in food packing materials. It must also neutralise and process the pesticides, fungicides and antibiotics which contaminate food and the environment; and any of the prescribed, recreational or social drugs. The liver never has a minute to itself. It produces bile, stores vitamins and minerals, sugar, blood and plasma proteins. It makes energy and heat, and breaks down, recycles or excretes hormones.

To protect liver cells

Silybum marianum (St Mary's thistle) seeds contain the most potent liver cell protective compounds known to exist.

Anti-oxidants, such as vitamins A, E and C, betacarotene and selenium.

Phosphatidyl choline, **or lecithin**, is a major component of healthy cell membranes. It protects liver cell membranes from damage from the continual attack of toxins and free radicals.

To improve bile flow

Bitter foods and herbs increase the flow of bile which is the vehicle for removing the substances broken down by liver cells.

To improve detoxification

Specific **herbs** can improve liver enzyme activity such as *Silybum marianum* (St Mary's thistle) and *Schizandra chinensis.* (More on these under Herbs, coming up.)

Sulphur compounds found in cabbage family vegetables, garlic, and dandelion can induce enzyme reactions in the liver which assist with detoxification. Brussels sprouts and cabbage, for example, can improve the breakdown and removal of some drugs.

An adequate **protein** intake is necessary to deal with some toxic materials.

Carbohydrates assist with detoxification pathways. Low-kilojoule diets may not provide enough carbohydrate for the liver to function as an organ of detoxification.

Minerals such as magnesium, calcium, zinc, copper and iron are essential components of many of the enzymes needed to drive detoxification pathways and arc also involved in biochemical reactions which help to prevent free radical damage in liver cells. Information pages on magnesium, calcium, zinc and iron are in the Minerals section of the Self Care chapter. Magnesium is a particularly good mineral because it helps with the symptoms of hormonal imbalance.

Eat foods which help the liver correctly process oestrogens, especially **methionine** found in beans, eggs, onions and garlic.

To help your liver function, eat some of these foods when you can: endive, chicory, silverbeet, radicchio, outer leaves of cos lettuce, mustard greens, dandelion leaf, dandelion root ('coffee'), grapefruit, and any other bitter-tasting, green leafy, vegie-typey thingies. In the herbal department, look for extracts from St Mary's thistle, gentian, barberry, centaury, hops and artichoke leaves.

PLANT OESTROGENS (PHYTO-OESTROGENS)

The oestrogens made in our bodies are called endogenous oestrogens. Some plants naturally contain components that are structurally similar to oestrogen and can have similar effects on the body. These are called plant oestrogens. They are also known as phyto-oestro-gens. (Pronounced fight-oh-east-roe jens.) Eating some phyto-oestrogens every day is a good idea. Positive research results are relevant for just eating phyto-oestrogens as part of a normal diet — there is no evidence to support getting into complicated regimes of weighing foods and taking long-term supplements.

What are phyto-oestrogens?

One of the first hints that hormones in plants could affect mammals came from the discovery that infertile sheep had been eating clover containing 'plant oestrogens'. Now, don't panic. This doesn't mean that if you eat clover-based honey you're infertile, or anything like that. If you've been going through a paddock or two of clover every week you might need to worry. (In more ways than one.)

Anyway, what we do now know, after researchers have ferreted around in laboratories, and a bit of trial and error, is that plant oestrogens are found in lots of growing things and that eating them can affect human health. Phyto-oestrogens we eat that can affect our health include isoflavonoids, coumestans and lignans; the triterpenoid and steroidal saponins, the phytosterols and the resor-cylic acid lactones, including zearalenone. All of them are naturally occurring compounds found in a large range of whole foods including grains, seeds (linseeds have lots of phyto-oestrogens but linseed oil doesn't, for example), legumes, and medicinal plants, as well as other common foods.

Foods with plant oestrogens

Isoflavones, especially soya beans and all other legumes; whole grains.

Coumestans, especially soya sprouts; and all other sprouted beans or legumes, split peas, mung beans.

Lignans, especially linseeds; and whole rye, buckwheat, millet, sesame and sunflower seeds, legumes and beans, whole grains.

Resorcylic acid lactones: oats, barley, rye, sesame seeds, wheat, and peas.

Steroidal saponins, especially real liquorice, and potato.

The effects of phyto-oestrogens

The effects of plant oestrogens on our hormones are pretty complicated. They can cause periods to get lighter and less frequent, reduce the incidence of oestrogen-dependent cancers, and help with menopausal symptoms, especially hot flushes.

Asian women who eat a traditional diet excrete higher amounts of endogenous oestrogen than women who eat a 'Western' diet, which some researchers believe accounts for their lower risk of breast cancer. Soya products consumed regularly in Asian countries contain high levels of phyto-oestrogens, and are said to be responsible for these positive effects, along with genes.

The lignans and some of the isoflavones require normal levels of bowel bacteria to turn them into the right stuff, so if you've taken, or are taking antibiotics, you probably won't get the full benefit. Eating yoghurt seems to help maintain the right bacteria.

How they work

Phyto-oestrogens share many of the same biological roles with oestrogens produced in the body. This is probably because phyto-oestrogens and body-made oestrogens are structurally similar, and both have the ability to interact with oestrogen receptors. We seem to need the phyto-oestrogens to balance our levels of oestrogens produced in the body throughout life.

According to lab tests, the oestrogenic effect of a phyto-oestrogen is estimated to range from around 160 to many thousands of times weaker than the body-made oestrogen oestradiol (pronounced eastro-die-al).

Before the menopause

Before menopause, the phyto-oestrogens we eat may help to protect against the 'proliferative effects' of too much oestrogen and reduce the incidence of related diseases like breast cancer, endometriosis and fibroids. Some diseases and cancers may develop because of the over-stimulating effect of too much oestrogen, but it's possible for phyto-oestrogens to prevent many of the more stimulatory oestrogens from occupying receptor sites: this is called competitive inhibition. Competitive inhibition is believed to be one of the ways that diets rich in isoflavonoids and lignans reduce the risk of oestrogen-dependent cancers. Tamoxifen, a drug which is used to treat breast cancer, is structurally related to the phyto-oestrogens.

The phyto-oestrogens are also capable of slowing down the production of extra, non- ovarian oestrogen produced in the fat tissues. As we've said, eating more soya products seems to lower the risk of breast cancer. This may be related to the phyto-oestrogens or be a result of many compounds acting together. There is evidence that eating phyto-oestrogens can help prevent cancer, but it isn't yet known whether eating phyto-oestrogens will help you if you already have an oestrogen-responsive breast cancer.

The isoflavonoids and lignans stimulate liver production of sex hormone binding globulin (SHBG). SHBG binds to the sex hormones, especially androgens and oestrogens, and acts as a carrier protein. When the major portion of these hormones are bound to SHBG in the blood, they are less available to bind to hormone-sensitive tissues. This is believed to be another way in which phyto-oestrogens lower the incidence of hormone-related diseases.

The symptoms of excess androgen production seen in polycystic ovarian syndrome (PCOS) and androgen disorders may be reduced by high levels of phyto-oestrogens because of the increase in SHBG. SHBG reduces the availability of androgens and may limit their masculinising effects.

Period regulation
Other more immediate benefits from phyto-oestrogens include lighter periods and longer menstrual cycles. They also reduce the risk of episodes of endometrial hyperplasia (too much cell production in the uterine lining).

Improved bone density

A new area of research is the potential for phyto-oestrogens to improve bone density. Positive results about humans are in the preliminary stages of research; however, positive benefits have been demonstrated for both dietary phyto-oestrogens and some phyto-oestrogen supplements.

After menopause

After menopause, the phyto-oestrogens have a mildly oestrogenic effect because they become more prevalent in a relatively oestrogen-poor environment. Recently Australian researchers found soya flour (high in phyto-oestrogens) decreased hot flushes by 40 per cent compared to 25 per cent in a wheat flour group (wheat flour is lower in phyto-oestrogens).

Getting your phyto-oestrogens

Increasing soya intake can be as easy as substituting low fat soy milk for ordinary milk and using soya flour in cooking. Tofu is very useful, and even 100 grams a day can reduce hot flushes and vaginal dryness. Dried or 'fresh' soya beans (you can buy them frozen in Asian food shops) can be added to soups and bean dishes. As little as 25 grams or about 2 heaped dessertspoons of ground linseeds per day can help to reduce symptoms of low oestrogen levels, including vaginal dryness. Linseeds contain lignans and can be used in cooking or ground and added to muesli, porridge, or drinks, like a smoothie. (The easiest way to grind seeds is in a coffee grinder you don't use for coffee beans. It's best to grind and eat them immediately so there's no chance of rancidity.) Don't buy pre-ground linseeds.

HERBS

Presumably one day a cavewoman realised it made more sense to put soothing herbs on a cut rather than rub in some gravel. Good one, Og.

Evidence that plants may have been used as medicines as early as sixty thousand years ago came from the discovery of the pollens of common plant medicines at the burial site of a Neanderthal man. Marshmallow, grape hyacinth, yarrow, ephedra — all in use today — were placed beside him, maybe as decorative offerings, or perhaps for his journey to the afterlife. (It's also possible that he died because the naughty boy didn't take his herbs, and he was used ever after as an example. Cave-parents would say things like, 'Remember what happened to Urp? So eat up all your yarrow and hyacinth or there'll be no mammoth for dessert.')

Virtually all peoples throughout the world have used some form of plant medicine. Those who still use herbal remedies seem to share common traits. Almost all cultures have specialists — individuals entrusted with the knowledge of specific plants who will pass on the information only to selected initiates. Many made sure there were specialists: Australian Aboriginal groups and other cultures have different men's and women's knowledge and use of medicines.

Over centuries, careful observation revealed that there were optimum times to pick plants and administer medicines according to the phases of the moon, seasons or times of day; and that some parts of the plant were more effective than others. It soon became clear that some plants were more effective when administered in certain ways. Gradually the doctoring and supply of herbs developed into recognised professions: the physician became the early doctor and the apothecary became the pharmacist.

The remnants of writings from the Arabs, Greeks, Romans and Egyptians survived to give a good indication of the practice of herbal medicine by the scholarly and educated. But much of the early practice of women's medicine was continued as a verbal herbal gerbil tradition. Sorry. There were no gerbils. Information was either passed on from one initiate to another by the priestesses and 'wise women' to be used in strict accordance with the current law; or in the case of the common and everyday remedies, passed on from mother to daughter or between friends. The sisterhood has always been abuzz with contraceptive hints.

Science and medicine have remained sceptical of the effectiveness of plants for contraceptive purposes although some cultures still use them. Rue is still used in a number of cultures in Latin America, and the common pea is believed by some people to be responsible for the low birth rate in Tibet. The seeds of Queen Anne's lace (*Daucas carota*) have been investigated for their contraceptive qualities and found to stop implantation of the embryo as well as inhibit the production of progesterone.

Don't bother trying herbal contraception — what was once common knowledge and passed on through word of mouth is temporarily lost to today's herbalist. And eating a lot of peas would probably give the rhythm method a run for its money in the unreliability stakes. The other herbs could just make you sick, or even a bit dead.

Over the past 50 years, herbal medicine in the West has changed its focus from the individual patient to what individual herbs will do to an individual disease. Detailed information is now available on the effects of many herbal medicines and it is possible to prescribe precisely for a number of complaints. Many doctors and surgeons are now recommending their patients also try natural remedies if they are appropriate, where a few years ago they might have dismissed them as 'unscientific mumbo jumbo'. Doctors in Europe and Japan are increasingly likely to prescribe herbal remedies themselves.

So if doctors are prescribing herbs, what's the point of having herbalists? First, herbalists can offer something special if they retain their traditional understanding that underlying disharmony causes the problem. In this way, the whole person is treated, and not just symptoms. A real natural practitioner will still focus on the individual, on why there is disease rather than what disease, and consider the vitality and constitutional type of the person along with the particular strain of bacteria or the results of a blood test.

And of course, professional herbalists are trained to know a lot more about the correct combinations, doses and species required for treatment. A doctor or naturopath untrained in herbs might well recommend a useless dose or another strain of a plant that isn't exactly right.

One of the fundamental beliefs of herbalism is that the body will want to repair itself. Herbs are ideal agents to support healing and the return of normal function because they are gentle and effective when properly prescribed. If the situation demands it, a combination of the two disciplines can lead to the best possible outcome.

How to take herbs

Many herbs are strong stuff, and their effects can be changed by the presence of other herbs or drugs you are taking. So it's very important to be aware of a few rules:

- Do not self-prescribe herbs, or take a herb because it worked for a friend.
- Find a trained herbalist with a specialty in your problem.
- If you are on any other medication, tell both your herbalist and your doctor exactly what you are taking.
- Follow the instructions carefully. This is just as important as when you are taking prescribed drugs.
- Never assume a herb is harmless or can be taken whenever you feel like it because it is 'natural'. Some herbs are naturally poisonous, toxic, otherwise dangerous, or useless in some combinations or doses and in certain situations.
- Any herb is unsafe in pregnancy in the wrong hands if taken at the wrong time, in the wrong dose or in the wrong combination.

Herb prescriptions are usually made up as mixtures in a bottle, looking somewhat like a cough mixture and tasting, in some cases, rather like eye of newt. Some herbalists will give you the roots, leaves and herbal extracts to boil up yourself on the stove. We recommend you don't have a hot date over on the same night, as the house is likely to smell somewhat startling. Some herbs and most supplements (like vitamins and minerals) are available in tablet form.

Herbs for women's trouble

There is a large range of the herbs used to treat 'women's' complaints — some of them have been used and modified for thousands of years. Others are providing new and contemporary possibilities. Modern science has more recently begun to support and extend the understandings of the uses of these herbs, through scientific testing and a more open mind.

None of these herbs may be prescribed by somebody without specialist training. Most of the herbs have lots and lots of other effects as well as gynaecological ones, and all these need to be taken into account when working out a prescription. For example, rue, an emmenagogue herb, has been used as an insecticide, a sedative, and a trial preparation with some promising results on multiple sclerosis symptoms.

The results of clinical trials on the herbs and their effects, doses, and information about how they must be prepared and prescribed by practitioners is outlined in Ruth's book, *Women, Hormones and the Menstrual Cycle*, published by Allen & Unwin.

Herbs affecting the hypothalamic-pituitary unit

A number of herbs are used for period problems related to a disturbance in the hypothalamic-pituitary department. These disorders can cause a wide range of complaints including heavy periods or no periods at all, irregular cycles and PMS.

Vitex agnus castus (chaste tree berries)

Vitex agnus castus is said to be a herb for the luteal phase (second half of the cycle) and can be useful for heaps of gynaecological complaints, especially ones which appear or get worse before the period. Many PMS symptoms, such as fluid retention and breast soreness improve with Vitex.

Latent hyperprolactinaemia (a result of changes in the activity of the hypothalamic–pituitary unit) causes problems such as PMS, disturbed menstrual cycle lengths, stopped ovulation and periods. Vitex seems capable of improving stopped periods, menstrual irregularities, and especially cyclic changes caused by latent hyperprolactinaemia.

Smaller doses of Vitex can also be used to promote breast milk especially in the first ten days after childbirth. Leading up to the menopause, it can be used to regulate the menstrual cycle by improving the regularity of ovulation.

Vitex must be prescribed by a trained practitioner familiar with its actions and contraindications. It should be started in the early part of the cycle, preferably before ovulation, and is usually given as a single dose in the morning. Dosage is important – too high or too low may make some conditions worse – and should be adjusted according to the problem treated, any additional symptoms, and your age.

Vitex should not be prescribed when hormonal preparations are used, including the Pill, HRT, or any of the common progestogen drugs such as Provera, Primulut, Duphaston and Danazol. It should be prescribed cautiously by a practitioner for women under 20, for whom the hypothalamic-pituitary-ovarian interplay is still fragile and easily disrupted. For full benefit, it is usually prescribed for between three and nine months.

Paeonia lactiflora (peony, Bai Shao)

In traditional Chinese medicine (TCM) three different types of peony are used – the white peony (*Paeonia lactiflora*), red peony (also usually from *Paeonia lactiflora*, but collected from wild plants and known as Chi Shao), and peony bark from *Paeonia suffruticosa* (Mu Dan Pi). 'Peony' indicates white peony/Bai Shao.

Paeonia lactiflora is effective in the treatment of PMS, polycystic ovarian syndrome (PCOS), hyperprolactinaemia, not ovulating, infertility, endometriosis and adenomyosis, androgen excess, breast soreness and menopausal symptoms. These conditions have at their core various hormonal irregularities which are influenced by peony, including elevated androgens, low progesterone, high or low oestrogen, and elevated prolactin.

Other peony-responsive conditions include period pain and uterine overactivity during pregnancy, low oestrogen levels and erratic ovulation and low progesterone levels. Peony-containing formulas can also be used to treat lowered rates of fertility due to androgen excess.

The two-herb formula, Liquorice and Peony Combination, reduces testosterone levels in women with PCOS and improves pregnancy rates. The luteinising hormone

(LH) to follicle stimulating hormone (FSH) ratio is also normalised. The same formula is also useful for the treatment of hyperprolactinaemia.

Complaints linked to relative oestrogen excess also respond well to peony-containing formulations, including adenomyosis and endometriosis, uterine fibroids and breast soreness. Peony is also used in association with liquorice for abdominal pain caused by muscle spasm.

Cimicifuga racemosa (black cohosh)

Cimicifuga racemosa is used for hot flushes and arthritic complaints in menopause and for delayed teenage periods caused by hormonal imbalance, especially when associated with stress. It contains hormonally active substances, one of which suppresses luteinising hormone (LH) after long-term use, and two of which have weak oestrogen-like effects. During menopause, it helps to reduce symptoms of vaginal dryness and irritation over time, and trials show it to be as effective as synthetic oestrogen.

It is helpful for younger women with menopausal symptoms caused by removal of their ovaries. And *Cimicifuga racemosa* can be used instead of HRT, as well as HRT, or as a treatment to 'wean' you off HRT. To come off HRT you take both *Cimicifuga racemosa* and HRT together until the herb has taken effect (usually 6–8 weeks), then stop the HRT. It is usually combined with other herbs so see a practitioner for best results.

The uterine tonics

The uterine tonics may be taken through the whole menstrual cycle and are usually prescribed as part of a formula if a complaint involves the uterus. These herbs are used to treat period pain because they are believed to regulate the muscular activity of the uterus and help kick-start contractions which are regular, rhythmic and more orderly. Uterine tonics are prescribed for uterine pain, for abnormal bleeding patterns, for prolapse, malposition or enlargement of the uterus, to help with some fertility problems and/or to regulate uterine tone until labour starts, help with a smooth delivery and regulate labour contractions. All uterine tonics should be used with care in the first trimester of pregnancy because of a slight possibility of miscarriage. It's best not to use any medication during the first three months of pregnancy unless absolutely necessary, and then only under expert supervision.

Rubus idaeus/strigosus (red raspberry leaf)
Traditionally, the herb was drunk as a tea for period pain and heavy periods, to prevent or relieve pregnancy-related nausea, to ease labour and to assist with breast milk production. The active constituents of raspberry leaves relax the uterine muscle and, surprisingly, also initiate contractions. It's not usually useful for period pain unless prescribed with specific other herbs. It's a good uterine tonic following surgery of the uterus, including removal of fibroids, termination of pregnancy or a curette.

Chamaelirium luteum (false unicorn root or helonias)
Helonias is used for no periods, heavy periods, irregular periods, period pain and to regulate the uterus. It is

recommended to prevent miscarriage. Another traditional use is to regulate ovarian function and problems which originate 'in the first half of the cycle'. It's threatened in the wild because of the increasing demands for collection and so its use should be restricted. *Paeonia lactiflora* or *Aletris farinosa* can be good substitutes.

Aletris farinosa (true unicorn root)

This is one of the best uterine tonics for women with a sense of pelvic heaviness or congestion, especially beneficial for women in their forties and fifties. It's used traditionally, in combination with spasmolytic herbs, to prevent miscarriage. There are conflicting reports on its actions, and it needs to be used in combination with other herbs. Like all the uterine tonics, *Aletris farinosa* is recommended for light or absent periods, periods which are too heavy or too frequent, for period pain and infertility, and for symptoms that accompany retroverted uterus.

Angelica sinensis (Dang Gui)

Dang Gui, *Aletris farinosa* and *Chamaelirium luteum* can sometimes be used interchangeably. Dang Gui can also improve blood circulation through heart muscle and is a 'blood tonic'. It is prescribed for pallor, weakness, dizziness, and dry skin; late, irregular or absent periods; pale period blood; weakness after the period, after giving birth or while breastfeeding; and period pain. Dang Gui can increase uterine tone, strengthen and order contractions, and relax the uterine muscle. It shouldn't be used in the first trimester of pregnancy unless prescribed by a trained herbalist as part of a traditional formula. Dang Gui works best when combined with *Paeonia lactiflora* and *Ligusticum wallichii*. For period pain that's worse with cold and associated with a slow start to periods, it's prescribed with *Cinnamomum*.

Caulophyllum thalictroides (blue cohosh)

Historically blue cohosh was used to prepare the uterus for labour, for period pain and for various 'inflammations' of the uterus. It's ideal as a uterine tonic for the last six weeks of pregnancy to improve the normal function of the uterus during labour. On the other hand, it is recommended to prevent miscarriages. The trick for successful use during pregnancy is getting the right combination with other herbs.

Spasmolytics: the uterus relaxers

The spasmolytics or anti-spasmodic herbs have a relaxing effect on the smooth muscle and can slow or regulate the rate of contractions in the uterus and in the bowel. Spasmolytics reduce spasm and calm uterine activity; reduce period pain which is colicky, crampy or contraction-like; calm the uterus in pregnancy and help prevent miscarriage and early labour. Anti-spasmodic herbs are used for crampy period pain and are more effective if given to stop the onset of spasm, rather than to treat pain that has already started. They should be started several days before the expected onset of the period. There's often no point taking anti-spasmodics through the whole cycle.

Viburnum opulus (cramp bark) and *V. prunifolium* (black haw)

These viburnums have similar therapeutic effects and are used to treat any condition associated with uterine spasm. *Viburnum prunifolium* has been extensively used to treat spasmodic period pain, prevent miscarriage, and to tone the uterus after fibroid removal. The use of these herbs in pregnancy should be left strictly to trained herbalists. They are usually prescribed for period pain with other spasmolytics and are best combined with Warming herbs such as *Cinnamomum* or *Zingiber* to offset stomach upsets and to improve their effect.

Ligusticum wallichii (Cnidium or Chuan Xiong)

Used to relax smooth muscle and against period pain and uterine overactivity. *Ligusticum wallichii* and *Angelica sinensis* are traditionally combined to treat period disorders. *Ligusticum wallichii* also shows promising results in preventing miscarriage and early labour.

Astringents: drying herbs

The uterine astringents are used to 'dry up' heavy periods and include *Trillium erectum*, *Equisetum arvense*, *Achillea millefolium*, *Tienchi ginseng*, *Capsella bursa-pastoris* and *Hydrastis canadensis*. The important astringents for heavy periods in adolescence are *Achillea millefolium* (yarrow), *Alchemilla vulgaris* (ladies mantle), *Capsella bursa-pastoris* (shepherd's purse) and *Geranium maculatum* (cranesbill).

The herbs are a large group of (usually) tannin-containing plants which reduce blood loss. This effect is seen on the stomach lining, the bowel wall, on the skin, and in the urinary, respiratory and reproductive tract. Long-term administration of tannin-rich plants can reduce the uptake of nutrients, and long-term, continuous use is not a good idea.

Achillea millefolium (yarrow)

Achillea millefolium is an important herb mostly used to reduce heavy periods. It can also help with stopped periods, or to relieve pain or act as a uterine stimulant to increase muscular tone and start a period. This is because it has a number of different effects on the uterine muscle, the sum total of which result in uterine stimulation without also causing spasm.

Alchemilla vulgaris (ladies mantle)

Used traditionally for heavy periods, as an emmenagogue and to promote contractions during labour. It can also be used to treat period pain and regulate the menstrual cycle. It is popular in Europe for teenage heavy periods. It's also recommended for heavy bleeding around menopause, and for urinary incontinence in post-menopausal women.

Hydrastis canadensis (golden seal)

Its main effect on excessive bleeding is believed to be due to its action on the capillaries. *Hydrastis canadensis* is commonly used with other herbs in a mix for heavy periods, particularly the uterine tonics as well as the tannin-containing herbs such as *Achillea millefolium* and *Geranium maculatum*. It must not be used in pregnancy.

Capsella bursa-pastoris (shepherd's purse)

Used for heavy periods of practically any origin (but an understanding of the cause must always come first). It combines well with *Trillium erectum* and *Hydrastis canadensis*, but this combination has a very strong taste and people hate it. Shepherd's purse should not be taken by anyone with hypothyroidism unless closely supervised.

Lamium album (white deadnettle)

Lamium album is popular for late or heavy periods caused by stress or nervous tension and is specifically used for a lack of uterine tone and bleeding between periods caused by hormonal irregularities. It's also useful for late, irregular and light periods related to weakness, nutritional deficiencies and overwork. As always, a diagnosis is a must before treatment is started.

Panax notoginseng (Tienchi ginseng)

Good for heavy bleeding caused by conditions such as fibroids, dysfunctional uterine bleeding and childbirth. It is usually prescribed only at the time of bleeding. Not to be used during pregnancy. Because it's so effective at stopping bleeding (but not treating the cause), it is absolutely essential that the reason for the heavy periods be identified before treatment or a serious condition may be masked. It's also useful for conditions with localised, congestive pain; and heavy and/or dark clotted menstrual blood, which may be accompanied by immobile abdominal masses.

These can accompany complaints such as fibroids, endometriosis and period pain with congestive pain. For these types of conditions, Tienchi might either be prescribed all month or just when pain occurs.

Trillium erectum (beth root)

Trillium erectum is used as an aid to labour and to stop bleeding, to be used in and after the third stage of a birth. It's also used in any situation where abnormal bleeding is a feature of a gynaecological complaint.

It is the best herb for women 30 to 50 years old with heavy periods because it also seems to regulate ovulation. Long-term use – between three and six months – is usually needed.

Calendula officinalis (marigold)

Calendula officinalis can be taken internally for the treatment of heavy periods and seems to play a role in bringing on late periods. It is also a circulatory stimulant and reduces pelvic congestion, effects which when combined with its antimicrobial properties make it ideal for pelvic infections and inflammation. It also has a reputation as a mild anti-spasmodic and is useful in the treatment of endometriosis.

Warming herbs

Warming herbs improve the action of the anti-spasmodic herbs, especially when the period pain is aggravated by cold, relieved by heat (the trusty hot-water bottle), or you have a tendency to 'feel the cold' easily.

Zingiber officinale (ginger)

The Warming properties of *Zingiber officinale* make it useful for period pain that is improved by the application of heat or warm drinks, and it has analgesic effects. The prostaglandin-inhibiting actions probably are also useful. It is also useful for nausea and vomiting with a period.

Premenstrual and menstrual migraines can be helped by *Zingiber officinale*, but it may aggravate menopausal flushing.

Warming herbs are best if taken hot. To make ginger tea, grate 2–4 centimetres of fresh root ginger, place in a saucepan with 1–2 cups of water, cover and bring slowly to the boil. Keep covered and simmer for about ten minutes. Strain, add honey to taste and sip while still hot. If possible, also have a warm bath. Other herbs can be taken at the same time.

Cinnamomum zeylanicum (cinnamon)

It's good for 'cold' period pain or pain accompanied by other symptoms such as localised pain, dark clotted period blood and immobile masses. It is often combined with *Angelica sinensis*, *Ligusticum wallichii* and/or *Paeonia lactiflora*. *Cinnamomum zeylanicum* can also reduce heavy periods.

Anodynes: the painkillers

The best-known anodyne herb is the opium poppy, now pharmaceutically manufactured as morphine, codeine and pethidine. Much weaker anodynes still in use by herbalists play a secondary role when treating the cause of the pain.

215

Corydalis ambigua (corydalis)

One of the strongest anodynes used in herbal medicine, this herb has an analgesic effect estimated to be I per cent that of opium. It is rarely used alone, usually being combined with anti-spasmodic herbs for best effects.

Corydalis ambigua is used to treat congestive or crampy period pain. It can stop heavy periods and accompanying severe pain. Not to be used in pregnancy.

Piscidia erythrina (Jamaican dogwood)

This particularly useful herb has anti-spasmodic and sedative effects which reduce period pain. Piscidia erythrina has a very low toxicity, even at high doses, but mustn't be taken in pregnancy.

Anemone pulsatilla (pulsatilla)

Used in painful and spasmodic conditions of the uterus, such as spasmodic period pain, and inflamed conditions of the genito-urinary tract including the pain of pelvic inflammatory disease (PID) and some types of cystitis. Anemone pulsatilla can be used for stopped periods caused by nervousness or stress. For period pain it's often combined with Viburnum opulus or V. prunifolium. The herb is an emmenagogue, and must not be taken in pregnancy. The fresh plant is poisonous and it must be taken as a precisely prescribed tincture.

Tanacetum parthenium (feverfew)

Can be used for women of all ages for period pain, recurrent premenstrual, mid-cycle or peri-menopausal migraines. It must be used all month as a preventative for best results. During labour, it's said to increase the frequency and regularity of contractions and relax a rigid cervix and is also traditionally used as an emmenagogue to bring on delayed periods. An oft-repeated caution that it causes mouth ulcers is only related to chewing the fresh leaf which may cause a type of contact dermatitis on sensitive skin — not usually a problem with tablets or tinctures.

Nervines

The nervine tonics can be used for either anxiety or depression and are seen to have a 'balancing effect'; the nervine sedatives are calming, and the nervine stimulants do what you'd expect — one of them is coffee. Nervines find a particular role in gynaecology in the treatment of premenstrual and peri-menopausal complaints, and as adjuncts to the treatment of period pain.

Hypericum perforatum (St John's wort)

Used for the treatment of mild to moderate anxiety and depression. It is especially useful during menopause and good for conditions where exhaustion and tension combine with hormonal problems. *Hypericum perforatum* extracts (infusions or fluid extracts) may produce photosensitisation if you're on a high dose or take the herb for a long time. Its use should be supervised.

Humulus lupulus (hops)

Hops is used for hot flushes, irregular periods with polycystic ovarian syndrome (PCOS), and flushing that accompanies stress, worry or insomnia. Hops, combined with *Cimicifuga racemosa*, is a useful treatment for PCOS perhaps because of their effect on luteinising hormone (LH) levels. It can also be used for spasmodic period pain.

Verbena officinalis (vervain)
Vervain can be used to treat spasmodic period pain and delayed periods, and to reduce the impact of menopausal symptoms.

Valeriana officinalis/edulis (valerian)
Herbal medicine's best-known sedative. It's used to boost the action of the spasmolytic herbs used in the treatment of period pain and is also good for sleeplessness.

Piper methysticum (kava)
It reduces the anxiety depression symptoms sometimes seen in association with menopause, and can also be used for PMS anxiety. Used in the Pacific region as part of religious ceremonies and in kava bars, where it is used like wine. Kava abuse has been reported in the Pacific and northern Australia, but this is linked with intakes more than ten times the recommended therapeutic dose used by herbalists.

Adaptogens: the tonics
Adaptogens are prescribed like an old-fashioned tonic when stress is high, or during convalescence from surgery or illness. Tonics are often helpful following childbirth, during lactation, or around menopause. Adaptogens are often prescribed with extra herbs specific to other complaints.

Eleuthrococcus senticosus (Siberian ginseng)

Useful for any type of stress or during convalescence. It can regulate stress-induced PMS symptoms; it is a useful general tonic after childbirth and following surgery; and it is one of the best adaptogens for the menopause, especially in combination with other herbs for low oestrogen symptoms. Excess coffee intake should be avoided when taking any kind of ginseng.

Panax ginseng (Korean ginseng)

Panax ginseng is one of the most commonly used adaptogens for stress and depression. It is believed to be more 'stimulating' and tends to have an uplifting effect which is usually noticed fairly quickly. It should not be taken with herbs which contain large amounts of caffeine or by heavy coffee drinkers, or by anyone with high blood pressure, acute asthma, or acute infections including viral infections. *Panax ginseng* can be useful around menopause or for convalescence and exhaustion. Long-term unsupervised use, however, is not a good idea. Two weeks on, two weeks off is a sensible course.

Codonopsis pilosula (codonopsis)

Codonopsis pilosula can be used if *Panax ginseng* is too stimulating, or if there's anxiety as well as fatigue.

Glycyrrhiza glabra (liquorice)

Glycyrrhiza glabra has very weak oestrogen-like effects and is sometimes self-prescribed for menopausal symptoms. This is a risky practice, except in the short term, because it can cause an elevation in blood pressure, fluid retention

219

and potassium depletion with prolonged use. Those who self-administer are usually unaware of these cautions. Some have even taken the lolly liquorice under the mistaken impression that it has the same properties as the unrelated herb. It can lower androgen levels, especially with peony.

Glycyrrhiza glabra is commonly used for coughs and dry mucous membranes, gastric ulcers and other gastro-intestinal complaints and to improve tolerance to a herbal formula. Its use should be restricted to less than six weeks unless closely supervised.

The bitters: liver herbs

It is the taste of bitterness that gives these herbs many of their therapeutic effects. The bitter taste on the tongue triggers a series of impulses which are carried by the nervous system and culminate in physiological and biochemical changes. Bitters medicine has the ability to improve your overall state by improving digestion, assimilation and (do you mind) evacuation (that's what it says here).

Taraxacum officinale (dandelion root)

Taraxacum officinale root is used as a general liver tonic and diuretic after debilitating illness or surgery; to improve liver function generally, and especially in conditions related to relative oestrogen excess such as endometriosis; or to protect the liver from the effects of hormonal preparations, including the Pill. It can be used after childbirth as a laxative and to increase milk flow.

It's advertised as dandelion root coffee. It tastes more like dirt than a cafe latte but it's good for you.

Berberis vulgaris (barberry)

A very useful liver herb for women with congestive period pain where the flow is slow to start, or where the pain is relieved when the flow commences. The flow is easier, redder and usually starts quickly and there's less heavy, dragging pain. *Berberis* is used for oestrogen-related conditions like endometriosis.

Silybum marianum (milk thistle or St Mary's thistle)

Silybum marianum is useful at any time that a liver dysfunction is a factor in a gynaecological problem. It is one of the best liver-protective agents known and is also a gentle laxative.

Bupleurum falcatum (bupleurum)

This is the most commonly used herb in Chinese medicine, used in four out of five traditional formulas. *Bupleurum falcatum* is prescribed for period problems accompanied by stress and worry, stopped periods, irregular periods, period pain and PMS. For these complaints, it is usually combined with *Paeonia lactiflora* and *Angelica sinensis*.

Diuretics

A diuretic is any substance that increases urine output. Some are only effective if the patient already has a diminished urine output, others can have effects which are comparable to drugs.

Herbal diuretics include celery juice, parsley, and dandelion leaf tea. You could try a vegetable juice with parsley and celery in it, or some herbal diuretic tablets, if your practitioner says it's a good idea.

Taraxacum officinale (dandelion leaf)
A very safe and effective diuretic that, unlike many diuretics, adds to the body's stores of potassium instead of depleting it. *Taraxacum officinale* leaf assists with the symptomatic relief of premenstrual fluid retention. To make dandelion leaf tea, add one or two teaspoons a cup, twice daily. You can mix it with peppermint tea, because it does taste a bit like grass clippings. Drink it in the morning.

Juniperus communis (juniper berries)
Juniperus communis has a reputation as a fertility control agent and an abortifacient. This herb should not be used in pregnancy by the untrained and should be used cautiously for any complaint. The injudicious use of juniper oil has caused death and so the oil is unavailable. The mild diuretic activity of *Juniperus communis* makes it a suitable premenstrual remedy especially in cases of urinary irritation or premenstrual low-grade urinary tract infections. The mild emmenagogic activity can also be useful to bring on a delayed period caused by hormonal irregularities, especially associated with discomfort and bloating. The cause of the hormone imbalance should always be treated.

Equisetum arvense (horsetail)

Equisetum arvense is a safe, gentle and well tolerated diuretic, even at high doses and during long-term use. For heavy periods, especially those accompanied by premenstrual fluid retention, it can be given throughout the cycle.

Self Care

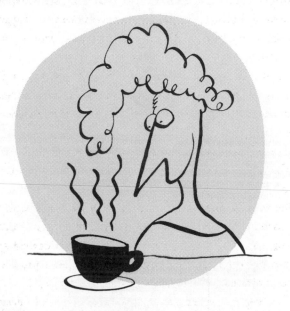

Caring for yourself is not about self-diagnosis or treatment without proper guidance. It does involve learning to recognise signs and symptoms to prevent illness. If you learn more about your body it will help you to recognise early signs of any change that may need attention.

Here are some important things to remember about looking after yourself:

- Get tested. Breast exams and cervical screening (Pap tests) are available from local doctors, women's clinics and Family Planning centres. You should have an internal pelvic examination every year to detect any changes in the pelvic structures, particularly the ovaries.

- Learn to 'listen' to your body. This doesn't mean a hippy-drippy psychic version of the stethoscope, it means if you really feel like there's something wrong, there probably is. Don't ignore warning signs and symptoms.

- Take prescriptions from doctors and natural therapists exactly as recommended, and make sure that each of your health care providers knows what the other ones are doing.

- Don't self-diagnose, don't prescribe yourself drugs or herbs, and don't wear your underpants on your head. You'll look stupid.

- Be as well informed as possible about any condition or disease you are dealing with. Don't just read one book, or one theory, or listen to one piece of advice. It can be tempting to fasten onto one reason or theory to explain everything, because it's simple.

- Be willing to accept that self care can only go so far with some conditions, and further or more complex treatment may be necessary.

- Remember that even if you are doing all the right things with your diet and lifestyle, you may still need to manage an illness in other ways. Don't be mad at yourself, just think how much worse it would be if you had a packet of Peter Stuyvesants and a Coke for breakfast every day.

EATING FOR HEALTH

About the closest most doctors get to asking about your diet is to say, 'Are you eating well?' To which you can reply, 'Oooh yes, doctor', meaning that you skip breakfast, have eight Tim Tams for lunch and usually eat the weight of a small Torana each evening, mostly from the food groups entitled 'lard' and 'utter crap'.

Natural therapists are more likely to pry into your eating habits and suggest some specific changes. Let's be frank: eating properly doesn't mean you'll never get sick, but it will make you healthier and less likely to get sick. And it means you recover more quickly. Not that we're the type to say, 'Oh, you've just had your leg amputated. Half a cup of dandelion tea a day and that'll grow right back in no time.'

Here's a 'top 20' of sensible suggestions for healthy eating. It's a general guide which you can use to introduce healthy changes to the way you eat. Don't try and change everything at once, don't regard the hints as a set of hard and fast rules and don't start faffing around the place weighing bits of food and stressing about whether you need another 76.4 grams of tofu before Thursday, or you'll bore yourself to death.

Remember that girls who haven't finished growing to their full height, and pregnant women, will need more of everything (well, you know, food, not bottles of gin) than the average adult woman.

20 GOOD-EATING HINTS

1. Eat varied and interesting food

We're not talking about sitting down to a bowl of chaff three times a day with half a mung bean for morning tea. Don't eat foods you hate just because 'they're good for you'. Lots of different kinds of food is the go. And relax. You're not going to explode if you have a chocolate bickie every now and then.

2. Drink plenty of fluids every day

Because otherwise you'll shrivel up like a dried apricot and blow away. Well, not quite. But you need at least 2 litres of water a day, and more when it's hot or you're exercising. By the time you have a dry mouth, dehydration has already started, so don't wait until you're really thirsty.

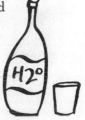

Fluids should be varied and should not come only from coffee, tea and fluffy duck cocktails. Two or three glasses of plain water, preferably filtered, throughout the day are essential. Fruit juices should be diluted because of their high sugar content.

3. Eat fresh and organic foods

Fresh is best — there are fewer preservatives, the food is less likely to be rancid, nutrient levels are higher and it tastes better. It's easier to see if fresh food has been spoiled or is old and past its 'use by' date. The closer you can get to the original source of the food, the better. This doesn't mean you have to go out and pick everything yourself, it means make sure your best pal is not the can-opener. Where possible, buy organic foods to minimise exposure to chemicals.

4. 'Therapeutic' diets are temporary

A therapeutic diet is prescribed with a particular goal — say, lowering cholesterol, improving anaemia, getting rid of thrush, or calming an irritable bowel. Therapeutic diets should only be used until the result is achieved, and always under the supervision of a health practitioner. Many of them don't contain the required nutrients, kilojoules or balance for extended use. If you react badly, go off it: therapeutic diets are not appropriate for all conditions or people.

5. Eat 5 to 7 different vegies and 3 fruits a day

Vegies and fruit contain a good range of vitamins, minerals, trace elements, essential fatty acids, antioxidants and fibre. Particular foods can also help to target particular problems. Cabbages and tomatoes reduce cancer risk; legumes contain plant oestrogens; bitter components flush the gall bladder; fruit pectin lowers cholesterol; and celery lowers blood pressure and reduces acid build-up in joints.

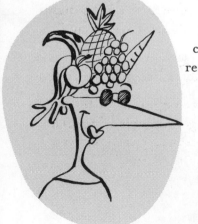

The old habit of 'a huge hunk of meat and three vegies boiled to death' should be abandoned with a sense of wild glee. To retain the most nutrients, it's best to cook vegies by steaming, stir-frying or baking. Every day you should eat from two to three different orange, red or yellow vegetables, a minimum of two green vegetables, and at least one of the cabbage family such as broccoli or cabbage – and some garlic or onion for their cancer-preventing and blood vessel protecting properties.

Fruit should be limited to three pieces a day because it doesn't seem to have the same energy-improving qualities of vegies (this may be because fruits are generally lower in minerals and higher in sugars). Fruit should preferably be eaten whole and not juiced, because juicing reduces the fibre content.

6. Main energy foods should be complex carbohydrates

Carbohydrates are energy foods which are eaten as whole foods like complex carbohydrates (such as brown instead of white rice) or as the more fatty and less useful refined carbohydrate like white bread. The main part of the diet should be based on complex carbohydrates from grains and legumes, dried beans and peas, nuts and seeds, soya products and some of the root vegies like potato, carrots and sweet potato. Common good energy foods include breakfast cereals and muesli, bread, rice, beans, tofu, pasta and potato.

Complex carbohydrates are high in fibre and many also contain plant oestrogens. They can lower blood cholesterol, stabilise blood sugar, regulate the bowel, reduce the appetite and ensure a good supply of regular energy. The slow energy release leads to greater stamina and fewer energy slumps. This is important for anyone troubled by blood sugar symptoms, and you there with premenstrual sugar cravings.

Carbo combos
Complex carbohydrates contain some of the amino acids which make up proteins and can be combined in a meal so that they become a substitute for animal protein. Carbohydrate-combining should be used by vegetarians to make sure that they get enough protein every day. The common combinations are:

- Grains with beans: tofu and rice (Asia), lentils and rice (India), tortilla and beans (Mexico).
- Grains and nuts: peanuts and rice (Southern Asia), nut butters and bread (bread-eating countries), rice and cashews (Asia).
- Beans and seeds: sesame seed paste and beans (Middle East).

Many people instinctively cook like this or follow traditional recipes which incorporate food combinations. Combining carbohydrates gives all of the energy benefits of protein, as well as the positive benefits of complex carbohydrates without a high animal fat intake.

7. Eat enough fibre
Eating more fibre can correct a blocked-up or farty bottom (known in the trade as bowel complaints), and reduce the incidence or severity of diabetes, gall stones and heart disease. A high-fibre diet lowers the risk rate of breast and colon cancer.

The best source of dietary fibre is from whole foods, but occasionally it may be necessary to use processed fibre

 230

products (like wheat bran, oat or rice bran), to effectively treat some diseases. Wheat bran, 'fibrous' vegetables (like celery and carrot), potato and other root vegies, tofu, legumes and linseed meal are all good sources of fibre.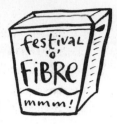

Fibre is sometimes included in therapeutic diets to achieve a specific outcome such as lowering of blood fats (cholesterol) and oestrogens; to reduce the incidence of gall bladder disease and colon cancer; for weight loss; or to treat constipation. Fibre is specifically important for women because it reduces the risk of oestrogen-dependent cancers, including breast cancer.

The recommended daily intake for fibre is 30 grams for an adult from whole foods and not as fibre-only breakfast cereals. This could be achieved by eating the following in the one day: five serves of wholegrain or legume products (such as two slices of bread, a cup of cooked beans, a cup of brown rice, and a cup of breakfast cereal) and five serves of different vegetables and three pieces of fruit.

8. Eat fewer 'bad fats' and more 'good fats'

Fat is the devil! It causes heart disease! It turns you into a hideous gargoyle! You'll get cholesterol problems and your head will fall off! And now they've invented a synthetic oil with no absorbable fat which causes 'anal leakage'. So what! It hasn't got any fat! Hmmm. It's just an inkling, but maybe it's time to get a bit less hysterical.

The fact is that if you cut out all fats you'll have more problems than when you started. There's good ones and bad ones. We all need a reasonable level of fats in our diet. They are essential for the production of sex and adrenal hormones, for the health of our skin and mucous membranes. When the right fats are eaten, they protect against high cholesterol and heart disease, skin and period problems and a whole lot else.

Bad fats

- An overall reduction of all fats is good.
- Cut down on saturated fats — they're in animal products (pork, beef, dairy products and lamb) and in the tropical oils (coconut and palm oils). Excessive saturated fat intake is linked to heart disease, obesity and an increased risk of some cancers.
- Cut down on the Omega-6 polyunsaturated fats. High levels of Omega-6 polyunsaturated fats are found in cooking oils and margarine.
- Avoid trans-fatty acids. These are in oils which are processed to become solid, like margarine and vegetable shortening. The high temperature process changes the oil molecule, and destroys essential fatty acids ('good fats'). Trans-fatty acids interfere with the production of the useful group of prostaglandins which prevent PMS, period pain and a heap of inflammatory problems.
- Look for 'contains hydrogenated fats' on labels and avoid it.
- Overall, too many fats, sugars, alcohol or carbohydrates are converted into triglycerides which increase

the risk of heart disease, kidney failure, high blood pressure and cancer.

- To reduce risk of heart disease, cholesterol-containing foods should be minimised, but the 'good fats' must be increased as well, to have the right effect. Cholesterol is used by the body to make hormones and other bits and pieces, so you shouldn't cut it out altogether. It is found in all animal fats but not vegetable fats. (The body makes its own cholesterol, partly from eating cholesterol, and partly as a response to eating other saturated fats.)

Good fats

To let the good fats do their work properly, you need to cut down on the bad fats, which can interfere with their work.

- Mono-unsaturated fats are the good vegetable oils to cook with and are more stable than polyunsaturated fats when they are exposed to heat, light or oxygen. Olive oil is the best-known mono-unsaturated oil and when used as a substitute for saturated fats, helps to lower cholesterol and reduce the risk of heart disease.
- Fatty acids are necessary for the normal function and development of most tissues including the kidney, liver, blood vessels, heart and brain. A deficiency leads to excessive scaliness of the skin, reduced growth rates and infertility in both males and females; and can also cause a greater susceptibility to infections, fragile red blood cells and difficulty in making prostaglandins.

Omega-3 fatty acids

The Omega-3 fatty acids are particular polyunsaturated fats. Suffice to say that we all need Omega-3 fatty acids, which are known as EPA (eicosapentaenoic acid) and DHA (docosahexaenoic acid). ALA (alpha linolenic acid) is an essential fatty acid which the body cannot make itself from other fatty acids.

To keep your prostaglandins in balance, and to control imbalance-related conditions, like period pain, some kinds of infertility, wound healing — all sorts of things — you need to regularly eat foods rich in Omega-3 fatty acids.

To make the right prostaglandins, you need to include these Omega-3s in your diet:

Linseeds or linseed (flax seed) oil These are very rich sources of ALA. You can take 1 to 2 tablespoons of ground linseeds a day. To help digestion and absorption, linseeds should be ground in a coffee grinder used only for seeds, never coffee (or mortar and pestle if you're feeling rustic), and can be sprinkled on muesli or tossed in a smoothie. They must be refrigerated in airtight containers or scoffed immediately after grinding. (Don't bother buying the pre-ground linseeds in packets at health food shops.) Alternatively, you could take 2 teaspoons of linseed/flax seed oil a day to be stored the same way. When served as recommended, linseed oil has 60 per cent ALA.

Other sources Pumpkin seeds (15 per cent ALA); canola oil (10 per cent); mustard seed oil (10 per cent); soya bean oil (7 to 9 per cent). Walnut oil also has moderate levels; and dark green leafy vegetables have small amounts. These fatty acids tend to go off and must be refrigerated in opaque bottles. No ALA oils should be cooked.

Oily fish The best fish to eat are cold-water and oilier fish. Include some of these fish in at least four meals a week. 'Oily' fish are often deep sea fish, where they've needed a bit of protection from the cold. If you can't buy fresh fish, get it in cans, although the benefits will be less obvious. Choose from: gemfish, blue mackerel, sea mullet, blue warehou, silver warehou, yellowtail kingfish, King George whiting, redfish, tuna, sardines, herring, pilchards, Atlantic salmon, silver trevally, luderick, ocean trout, blue eye, golden perch, blue grenadier, and rainbow trout.

Fish oil supplements are usually capsules which include 18 per cent EPA and 12 per cent DHA and are made from fish oils or fish liver oils. Cod liver and halibut liver oils, however, also contain vitamins A and D, which means that they are no good for the long term at large doses. (It's dangerous to take vitamin A supplements if you're pregnant.) Fish oils have a long list of therapeutic effects which includes reducing heart disease; reducing arthritic inflammation; and an improvement in allergy-related conditions such as asthma and eczema.

Omega-6 fatty acids
Linoleic acid Eat some of this when you can. There may be positive effects on infertility linked to endometriosis and in reducing heavy periods. Linoleic acid is found in seed and vegetable oils, as well as most nuts, and organ

meats. Coconut oil and dairy products contain very low levels of linoleic acid. Although the levels are low compared to seeds, any dark green vegetable is a source of linoleic acid. Linoleic acid is an essential fatty acid. Essential, in this case, merely means that you must eat them because the body won't manufacture them by itself.

There's lots of linoleic acid in seed oils: safflower oil (75 per cent); sunflower oil (60 to 70 per cent); walnut oil (60 per cent); corn oil (55 per cent); soya bean oil (50 per cent); peanut oil (35 per cent) and olive oil (8 per cent).

Evening primrose oil, blackcurrant seed oil and borage seed oil are also rich sources of linoleic acid.

Gamma-linolenic acid Gamma-linolenic acid (GLA) is the building block from which the body makes the prostaglandins that reduce inflammation, stop pain and activate the immune system. GLA is found in the oils of evening primrose, blackcurrant, safflower, sunflower, hemp, soybean, pumpkin seed, borage seed and walnut. These seed oils have been shown to reduce sore breasts and the severity of other PMS symptoms.

Evening primrose, star flower oil and blackcurrant seed oil are available as capsules which contain beneficial amounts of GLAs as well as linoleic acid.

Cooking and storing hints for oils

- Mono-unsaturated fats are the best oils for cooking. Pour them into a pan that's already hot to reduce heating time. Never re-use oils.
- Don't cook in other oils. Heating induces irreversible changes to many oils which leads to oxidation or free

radical formation. Foods can be cooked in just a little water, or even 'dry fried' in a non-stick pan. Fish, eggs and vegetables can be poached in water, or a fruit or vegetable puree, and fish and vegetables can be baked rather than roasted in oil.

· Add oils to food after cooking as salad dressings or sauces.

· Eat more cold-pressed oils of linseed, safflower and canola as tablespoon doses once or twice a day or added to a seed breakfast or muesli, used in salad dressings, poured onto cooked food or mixed with yoghurt in a ratio of about one part oil to five parts yoghurt.

· Make your own spreads with avocado, tahini, yoghurt, chickpeas, nut butters or vegetable-based dips instead of margarine or butter.

· Buy oils manufactured without damage to the goodies ('cold-pressed', 'unrefined' or 'mechanically extracted') and in opaque glass bottles. All oils and oil-containing foods should be refrigerated. Otherwise they have a habit of going off.

9. Eat dairy products in moderation

Many people are sensitive to dairy products, or at least some aspects of them, and some natural therapists recommend that they not be eaten at all, while dietitians see the enormous potential for nutrients, especially calcium, and recommend a high intake. What's going on? Are they good for us or what? Well, they're okay, if you eat the low-fat varieties, unless you have a dairy intolerance, and even then, you probably can eat yoghurt.

Don't drink milk with lactose if you're intolerant.

237

Here's a simple test: somebody comes up and asks you the time, do you strike them repeatedly with your handbag? That is very intolerant. (Seriously, any food intolerance or allergy should be appropriately diagnosed.) Yoghurt is an important food. It is easily digestible, provides good bacteria which makes the gut work properly, has more calcium than milk, and may help to reduce the risk of breast and other oestrogen-dependent cancers. It is also well tolerated by those with a dairy or lactose intolerance.

Read the label to make sure a yoghurt has live cultures; many of the snack-type yoghurts don't, especially the flavoured and 'fruit yoghurts'. Get low-fat, no-sugar brands.

Don't forget bones need magnesium too, if calcium is to be properly retained, and dairy foods don't have much magnesium.

10. Eat plant oestrogens

Plant oestrogens, also known as phyto-oestrogens, are structurally similar to animal oestrogen and are found in a large number of common foods and medicinal plants. Eating plant oestrogens is associated with a reduced incidence of oestrogen-related disease such as endometriosis, and breast and endometrial cancer. A full explanation of plant oestrogens is in the previous Natural Therapies chapter.

11. Eat enough protein regularly

When people go on 'healthy' or 'weight-loss' diets, they often drastically reduce or stop most of their protein

 238

intake. Protein is found in animal products such as meat, eggs, fish, milk and cheese, and also in the vegetable proteins such as tofu. Neither type is better or worse, unless you're a vegetarian.

Vegetarians (lacto-ovo), for example, can obtain protein from eating vegetable proteins, dairy products and eggs; vegans get it from eating combinations of vegetables. It's harder to get iron, and for the vegan, to get vitamin B12 as well. The advantage of being a vegetarian is a lower intake of fat and less likelihood of developing many of the chronic degenerative diseases; the disadvantage is a tendency to anaemia and fatigue.

Meat-eaters have an advantage when it comes to iron intake. Iron in meat is easier to absorb and it is present in much greater quantities. Animal protein is also of a better quality and meat-eaters can have a more relaxed attitude to nutrient intake and still maintain energy levels. On the down side, eating meat increases the intake of saturated fats and the risk of a number of diseases, such as heart disease and cancer. Deep sea fish is better because it contains high levels of essential fatty acids as well as protein. This means you have to ask the fishmonger if the fish is from the deep sea. Or there's a list of oily fish under Bad Fats and Good Fats, number 8 in this list.

For those who do eat meat, protein can come from (preferably chemical-free) lean, red meat in small quantities, some free-range chicken without the skin, plenty of fish, no more than three eggs a week and low-fat dairy products. You should have animal proteins at only one meal a day. The protein in other meals should come from properly combined vegetable sources. How to combine

239

them is explained in the dietary guidelines for hypogly-caemia, pages 184–8.

It's kind of complicated, but on average, women over 20 should eat about 45–55 grams of protein each day. If you're between the ages of 11 and 20 you need to add another 10–50 grams to that. Here are some levels of protein in food:

100 grams of meat	20–25 grams
100 grams of seafood	15–20 grams
1 cup beans/legumes	7.5–15 grams
1 cup whole grains	5–12 grams
1 cup milk or yoghurt	8 grams
1 egg	6 grams
30 grams of cheese	6–8 grams
1 cup vegies or fruit	2–4 grams

12. Know your minerals
The key ones for women are in the next section, aston-ishingly enough entitled 'Minerals'.

13. Eat foods in season
Apart from the ludicrous price of foods that are out of season or imported (Darling, how marvellous! These July raspberries are only $6000 a punnet!) there's another reason to buy what's locally available at the right time of year.

All fruits and vegetables can be assigned with certain qualities in the same way that medicinal herbs are. Summer foods are generally juicy and light, winter foods tend to be dense and compact with lots of carbohydrate and protein. In summer, moist, easily digested raw foods make sense, but in winter they don't provide enough carbohydrate to counterbalance the energy expenditure needed to stay warm.

Winter foods should be mainly beans, legumes and root vegetables; salads can be made from root vegetables and cabbage. These are Warming and comforting foods on a cold winter's day.

Most summer fruits and vegetables have Cooling properties — melons are particularly Cooling while bananas, which tend to be dense and compact, are Warming. Eat stuff that seems instinctively right for that time of the year.

14. Vary the flavours

There are five main flavours in the diet: bitter, sweet, sour, salty and spicy or pungent. Australians traditionally rely heavily on the sweet and salty flavours, but other cultures include all or most of the flavours in their cooking as a matter of course — Thai food, for example, is cooked with the addition of salty, sweet, spicy and sour flavours.

Each of the flavours has subtle effects on digestion and health.

Bitter

Bitter foods improve digestion and bowel function by stimulating the bile flow. Bitter green vegetables and radicchio, chicory, dandelion leaves and silverbeet are often included in the European diet to aid digestion. (Spinach is not a 'bitter' because it doesn't taste bitter.) Grapefruit is sour and bitter, and the old practice of having half a grapefruit before a fatty breakfast such as bacon and eggs makes a lot of sense. (Almost as much as not eating the fatty breakfast every morning.) Dandelion coffee is a gentle and effective bitter that is available as a beverage. (It is available as a beverage that tastes like bat wee, if you asked one of the authors of this book, but we shall draw a tactful veil over this fact.)

Spicy

Warming spices in the diet improve sluggish digestion and are particularly useful for complaints of the upper gastrointestinal tract such as nausea, burping and indigestion.

Ginger, cardamom, cumin and coriander are all useful – ginger tea is particularly helpful for nausea. (Cut two or three bits of fresh knobbly ginger root, about 2 centimetres long, throw them in a teapot, add boiling water and let it steep for a couple of minutes.) These spices can be brewed in ordinary black tea to assist with digestion. Warming spices are useful for those who feel cold, have difficulties with cold weather, or catch colds easily.

Sour

Sour foods are drying and can be used to stop snuffy noses. For some people, sweet foods cause phlegm or catarrh and sour foods can reverse the process. Many sour foods, such as citrus fruit, are useful to protect the mucous membranes from infections. Sour foods also aid digestion.

15. Don't stuff yourself silly

Overeating (to be perfectly obvious) is linked to obesity and a shorter life expectancy. The digestive tract is chronically overburdened and the incidence of gall bladder disease increases. The heart has to work harder and the risk of high blood pressure also increases.

16. Don't argue with your food

Eat foods which agree with you. Listen to your body and act accordingly. Some common diets cause obvious problems in some people, such as abdominal upsets, diarrhoea, or fatigue. And sometimes your body decides it used to like something but now it's gone right off it.

Raw food diets can be a problem, for example, because raw food is quite difficult to digest. Bloating, wind or even diarrhoea can lead to a depletion of nutrients and ill health. Trading one health problem (for example, shocking wind) for another (like being overweight) doesn't make sense.

17. Limit sugar and salt

Sugar

All types of sugar should be minimised, including brown and unrefined sugars; as well as the foods which are prepared with sugar and processed food with added sugar (this includes stuff like tinned beans, even).

Salt

Salt intake is associated with high blood pressure and increases the excretion of minerals in the urine. Most sodium (salt) enters the diet in most manufactured foods, not through adding salt during cooking or at the table. Salt should be limited to around 3–5 grams daily.

18. Limit caffeine

Caffeine-containing drinks contain highly active substances known as xanthines. (Xanthines, while sounding like a girlfriend of Xena, Warrior Princess, are actually alkaloids which have diverse effects in the body.)

Caffeine is in coffee, tea, cocoa and chocolate. Caffeine increases anxiety, aggravates insomnia, helps to waste minerals and increases blood pressure. Excessive caffeine intake is also linked with a number of common gynaecological conditions including endometriosis, fibroids, PMS and benign breast disease. Caffeine has also been shown to lower fertility.

Gynaecological problems have been associated with the equivalent of two cups of coffee or four cups of tea every day. 'Plunger' coffee has the least harmful effects. Boiled coffee should be completely avoided if there are problems with high cholesterol levels.

19. Cut down on alcohol

Women are more affected by alcohol for longer periods of time than men. Women have a lower body water content and so alcohol is less diluted. They also metabolise (break down) alcohol more slowly because they have a smaller liver cell mass than men.

This is why there are different government health warnings for women and men. Two standard alcoholic drinks in less than an hour will take a woman to the legal

 244

blood alcohol limit for driving, but this figure may be influenced by hormonal fluctuations of the menstrual cycle (around the period and ovulation, alcohol is thought to be metabolised more slowly), by cigarette smoking and by diet.

Excess alcohol consumption has been linked to cancers, hypertension, heart disease, foetal abnormalities, and liver disease. A host of other more subtle health problems are caused or aggravated by alcohol. Some are caused by depletion of minerals such as calcium, magnesium, potassium and zinc, and vitamins A, C and the B complex, especially BI. The National Health and Medical Research Council have made the following recommendations for women:

- Women should limit drinking to two standard drinks or 20 grams of absolute alcohol per day and have two or three alcohol-free days a week to give the liver some recovery time.
- More than two drinks a day or 14 drinks a week is officially considered dangerous. Any more than that and you're officially damaging yourself.
- Don't drink at all if you're pregnant.

Also, if you do get legless drunk, don't go for the 'hair of the dog' and start all over again. Give your body free time to get over it: about two days between drinks is recommended.

20. Eat more serenely

A common cause of digestive problems and poor nutrient uptake, is the practice of eating in the car, watching TV or on the run. Meal times need to be a little sacred; a

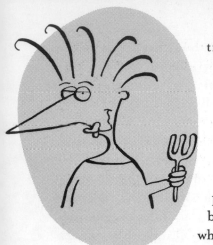

time set aside to think about food, be with family, friends or self. Taking time to chew food thoroughly is an essential beginning to good digestion. Avoid unnecessary argument or conflict and try not to eat when upset or in pain. If possible wait until you feel better. Most importantly, enjoy what you are eating. If you happen to eat some junk food, enjoy it, then get on with wholesome eating.

MINERALS

It is better to get all minerals from food, but if this isn't possible (as opposed to just inconvenient) you can take supplements. Always check with your health practitioner for acceptable doses for you.

Zinc
Most women don't get enough zinc — especially during the teenage years.

Some possible symptoms of zinc deficiency
Slow growth; infertility/delayed sexual maturation; hair loss; skin conditions of various kinds; diarrhoea; immune deficiencies; behavioural and sleep disturbances; night blindness; impaired taste and smell; white spots on finger-nails; delayed wound healing; post-op complications;

dandruff; impaired glucose tolerance; connective tissue disease; reduced appetite.

Zinc deficiency can be caused by
Anorexia nervosa, fad diets, 'weight-loss' diets; exclusion diets for food allergies; a strict vegetarian diet; restricted protein diets; long-term intravenous therapy or tube feeding through the nose; alcoholism.

Zinc absorption may be hampered by
High-fibre diets; iron tablets; coeliac disease (gluten intolerance); food allergies; low or absent gastric acid levels; alcoholic cirrhosis; a dicky pancreas.

You need extra zinc if you're
- going through puberty or a growth spurt
- pregnant or breastfeeding
- taking diurctics
- on the drug penicillamine, a detoxifying drug
- suffering from psoriasis, exfoliative dermatitis, or excessive sweating
- troubled by intestinal parasites or hookworm
- drinking too much grog
- suffering from liver disease including viral hepatitis
- prone to chronic diarrhoea and ileostomy fluid loss
- recovering from surgery or trauma
- diagnosed with cancer

Recommended daily allowance
12—15 milligrams a day for women

Good sources of zinc

This chart shows how many milligrams of zinc are in 100 grams of food.

Fresh oysters (as if you'd be having those every day)	45–75	Peanuts	3
		Sardines	3
Wheat bran	16	Dark chicken meat	2.85
Wheat germ	13	Walnuts	2.25
Dried ginger root	7	Wholewheat bread	1.65
Brazil nuts	7	Prawns	1.15
Red meats	4.5–8.5	Whole egg	1.10
Parmesan cheese	4	Non-fat cow milk	0.75
Dried peas	4	Porridge	0.5
Hazelnuts	3.5	Raw carrots	0.5

Iron

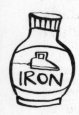

Iron requirements for women are around 80 per cent higher than for men. It is estimated that iron deficiency is the most common nutritional disease worldwide and that more than half of all women consume less than the recommended amount of 10–15 milligrams a day.

Those at most risk of iron deficiency

Pregnant women; women with heavy periods; children; vegetarians; serial dieters; people on strict exclusion diets; people with low gastric acid levels, such as after stomach surgery and with ageing; people with malnutrition.

Iron deficiency or anaemia?

Iron is stored in the body in red blood cells, the liver, bone marrow, spleen, muscles and in the serum. A test for anaemia will determine only whether there is a depletion of iron stored in the red blood cells (the haemoglobin level), but not whether iron levels are high enough in the rest of the body.

The symptoms of iron deficiency can happen before the red blood cells become depleted of iron. Many people are iron deficient even though their haemoglobin is normal. For this reason, many doctors now order a blood test to check iron stores in the plasma as well as the haemoglobin levels.

Symptoms of anaemia

Red blood cells need iron to be able to carry oxygen around the body. When that isn't around, anaemia symptoms happen, including poor stamina; shortness of breath on exertion; unreasonable limb fatigue and dizziness. Other symptoms seem to be related to the lack of iron in the serum, called iron deficiency.

Symptoms of iron deficiency

A red sore tongue and cracks in the corners of the mouth; excess hair loss; concave finger nails; reduced resistance to infection; poor digestion caused by low gastric acid levels. (Iron deficiency can cause decreased production of gastric acid and can be caused by it – a vicious circle.) Some people with iron deficiency have a strong desire to chew ice.

In children, symptoms include not thriving; slow learning; reduced infection resistance and poor appetite.

How to improve iron absorption

Apart from increasing the amount of available iron in the diet, there are a number of other ways to increase iron levels:

- Eat vitamin C rich foods, particularly when consuming foods high in iron.
- Add acidic dressings, such as lemon juice and vinegar, to iron-rich foods. This is a common southern Mediterranean practice, where there is a high incidence of inherited anaemia and the traditional diet contains little red meat.
- Eat bitter vegetables or fruit before or during the meal to increase the flow of gastric acid which will in turn improve the absorption of minerals. Alcoholic aperitifs, grapefruit, Swedish bitters and bitter green vegetables can all be used. Bitter vegetables are best because they usually contain iron as well as stimulating its absorption.
- When low gastric acid levels are accompanied by iron deficiency, taking iron may improve both.
- Avoid tea (especially black tea) or coffee until the iron deficiency improves. The tannin in tea binds with iron making it difficult to absorb.
- Coffee also reduces absorption, especially if taken with or after a meal, but not when taken more than one hour before eating.
- Definitely don't take iron tablets with a cup of tea or coffee.

Diagnosing low iron stores

Iron deficiency causes the symptoms described above and should respond to a low-dose iron supplement within a few weeks. Iron should not be taken unnecessarily as it will accumulate in the body and may become toxic. If symptoms do not respond, seek advice and ask for a blood test which evaluates serum iron levels.

Recommended daily allowance

10–15 milligrams a day for women

Good sources of iron

This chart shows how many milligrams of iron are in 100 grams of food.

Meat, fish and eggs

Mussels	7.7	Oysters	6.0
Lean beef	3.4	Lean lamb	2.7
Sardines	2.4	Eggs	2.0
Dark chicken meat	1.9	Lean pork	1.3
Light chicken meat	0.6	Cod	0.4

Grains

Special K	20.0	Wheat bran	12.9
All Bran	12.0	Wheat germ	10.0
Soya flour	9.1	Weetbix	7.6
Raw oatmeal	4.1	Whole wheat flour	4.0
Rye biscuits	3.7	Whole wheat bread	2.5
White bread	1.7		

Legumes and vegetables

Raw parsley	8.0	Spinach	3.4
Silverbeet	3.0	Haricot beans	2.5
Lentils	2.4	Leeks	2.0
Spring onions	1.2	Peas	1.2

Continued over page

Iron sources continued

Broccoli	1.0	Raw mushrooms	1.0
Lettuce	0.9	Jacket potatoes	0.6

Fruits

Dried peaches	6.8	Dried figs	4.2
Dried apricots	4.1	Prunes	2.9
Sultanas	1.8	Currants	1.8
Raisins	1.6	Dates	1.6
Avocado	1.5	Stewed prunes	1.4
Raspberries	1.2	Fresh apricots	0.4

Other

Yeast	20.0	Almonds	4.2
Brazil nuts	2.8	Walnuts	2.4
Peanuts	2.0	Hazelnuts	1.1

Magnesium

Magnesium is vital for the maintenance of bone density, the prevention of heart attacks and the functioning of all muscles. Magnesium is a crucial female mineral, but never seems to get the sexy telly ads, probably because calcium has a dairy corporation behind it, and the beef industry likes to bang on about iron.

Bones

Magnesium is almost as important for bone health as calcium. It improves the absorption of calcium from food and increases its retention in the body. A high intake of calcium inhibits the absorption of magnesium. Foods traditionally thought of as being useful for bone density, such as dairy products, are also relatively low in magnesium (a cup of milk contains 290 milligrams of calcium, but only 35 milligrams of magnesium) which raises doubts about the suitability of large intakes of dairy products for bone health. Magnesium, either alone or with calcium, offsets the usual overnight bone mineral loss.

The heart
Magnesium protects the heart muscle from getting overexcited which can cause irregularities in the heart beat.

PMS
Magnesium and vitamin B6 can help alter the hormone levels and protect against PMS.

Signs and symptoms of magnesium deficiency
Weakness and/or tiredness; poor muscle co-ordination; premenstrual symptoms; apathy; insomnia, hyperactivity; susceptibility to toxic effects of the drug digoxin; abnormalities of the heart's rhythm, an abnormal reading on an electrocardiograph (ECG) which traces heart activity; muscle cramps; grimaces, tremors of the tongue, 'flickering' eyelids; loss of appetite, nausea, constipation; confusion, disorientation and memory impairment, learning disabilities; vertigo; difficulty swallowing or throat constriction.

Obviously these symptoms can have other serious causes, but when no obvious cause can be found, improved magnesium intake may help.

Recommended daily allowance
The recommended daily intake for magnesium is 400–800 milligrams for women.

Good sources of magnesium

This chart shows how many milligrams of magnesium are in 100 grams of food.

Grains

Wheat bran*	520	Wheat germ	300
Whole wheat flour	140	Porridge	110
Muesli	100	Rye flour	92
White flour	36		

Seafood

Prawns	110

Vegetables

Beet tops	106	Silverbeet	65
Spinach	59	Raw parsley	52
Beans	35	Green peas	33
Broccoli	24	Beetroot	23

Beans and nuts

Brazil nuts	410	Soya flour	290
Almonds	260	Peanuts	180
Walnuts	130		

Fruits

Dried figs	92	Dried apricots	65
Avocado	30	Banana	20
Grapefruit juice	18		

* Foods that are rich in magnesium, such as bran, may not provide the best source of minerals. Magnesium can become bound to the phytates in bran which reduce absorption. Whole foods from a wide variety of sources is the best way to attain a good intake of easily absorbed magnesium.

Calcium

You can see below that the recommended daily allowance (RDA) varies depending on your age. If you are not getting enough calcium, you can either increase the number of calcium-rich foods, or take a supplement. To maintain the bone density to prevent osteoporosis you need to keep up a high calcium intake before, during and after the menopause. Post-menopausal women should consume 4–5 serves of calcium-rich foods in order to obtain enough calcium, preferably from different sources. In other words, don't just eat a vat of yoghurt every day.

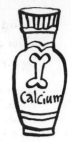

Recommended daily allowances
Babies: 350 550 milligrams
Kids aged 1 to 10: 800 milligrams
Teenagers: 1200 milligrams
Young women aged 20 to 35: 800–1000 milligrams
Pregnant/ breastfeeding women: 1500 milligrams
Women more than 35 years old: 1000 milligrams
After the menopause: 1500 milligrams

Low-kilojoule calcium sources
Girls going through the growth spurt of their teenage years who are exercising regularly shouldn't worry about eating whole-fat dairy products.

Others might like to consider these low-fat sources. All these low-kilojoule food sources have 300 milligrams of calcium:

$1^{1}/_{4}$ cups of cooked spinach or other greens; 2 cups cooked broccoli; 1 cup Physical milk; $^{2}/_{3}$ cup plain low-fat yoghurt; $^{1}/_{4}$ cup grated parmesan; 50 grams Swiss or cheddar cheese; $1^{1}/_{2}$ cups whole milk; $1^{1}/_{4}$ cups plain yoghurt; 200 grams tofu; 1 can sardines; 300 grams tinned salmon; 2 cups low-fat cottage cheese.

Good sources of calcium

This chart shows how many milligrams of calcium are in 100 grams of food.

Dairy products

Skim milk powder (dry)	1190	Goat's milk	130
Whole milk powder (dry)	900	Skimmed cow's milk	123
Whey powder	645	Buttermilk	115
Physical milk 100 ml	205	Cow's milk whole	115
Yoghurt—cow's	180	Human milk	30
Rev milk 100 ml	150		

Cheese

Parmesan	1091	Camembert (30% fat)	600
Gruyere	1000	Danish Blue	580
Mozzarella	817	Blue (50% fat)	540
Cheddar	810	Camembert (60% fat)	400
Gouda	810	Fetta	353
Edam (30% fat)	800	Ricotta	223
Edam (45% fat)	678	Cottage (low-fat)	77
Gorgonzola	612	Cottage	67

Eggs   56

Fish

Whitebait	860	Scallops	120
Sardines (canned)	550	Salmon (canned)	100

Soya products

Soya milk (dry)	330	Tofu	170
Soya grits	255	So Good soy milk	116
Dried soya beans	225	Vita Soy soy milk	32
Soya flour, full fat	210		

Nuts

Almonds	250	Walnuts	60
Brazil	180	Macadamia	50
Pistachio	136	Hazelnuts	45
Pecan	75	Peanut butter	35
Peanuts (fresh)	60	Cashews	30

Seeds

Unhulled sesame seeds	1160	Sunflower seeds	98
Linseeds	271	Pumpkin seeds	52
Hulled sesame seeds	110		

Grains and cereals

White flour	350	Wheat germ	69
Muesli (depends on brand)	200	Wheat crispbread	60
Wheat flour (white or brown)	150	Porridge	55
Wheat bran	110	Rye crispbread	50
Bread (brown or white)	100	Brown rice	33
All Bran	75	Weetbix	33
Rice bran	69		

Meat   10–20

Legumes (cooked)

Navy beans	95	Lentils	50
Chickpeas	70	Black-eyed beans	40
Kidney beans	70	Split peas	22

Sprouts

Alfalfa sprouts	28	Lentil sprouts	12
Mung bean sprouts	20		

Vegetables

Parsley	260	Onions	135
Watercress	190	Spinach	135
Dandelion greens	185	Broccoli	125
Spring onions	140	Silverbeet	115

Fruits

Dried figs	260	Rhubarb (stewed)	93
Lemons	110	Orange juice (100 ml)	60
Lemon juice (100 ml)	8	Blackberries	60
Other fruit except dried	10–50		

Other

Kelp	1095	Carob powder	355
Crude molasses	654	Brewers' yeast	210
Torula yeast	425		

What Now?

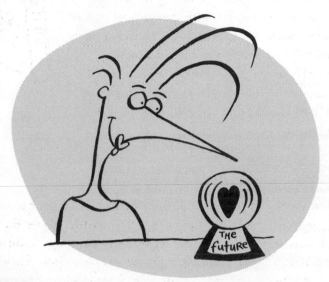

BOOKS

Endometriosis: Natural and Medical Solutions by Ruth Trickey and Kaz Cooke, Allen & Unwin, 2002. All the stuff you need to read about having endo and dealing with it — medically, with natural therapies, and self care. A sister book of this one.

Women's Trouble by Ruth Trickey and Kaz Cooke, Allen & Unwin, 1997. The mother of this book — much more detail about hormones, different conditions and options for treatment — be careful you don't spend money unnecessarily — there may be a lot of overlap on information about your condition already in this book.

The Curse by Karen Houppert, Allen & Unwin, Sydney 1999. An informative and political examination of how women are taught to be ashamed and secretive about periods. If you have a lot of trouble with periods you may quarrel with the 'periods are natural and wonderful' message but it's still a fascinating story about 'the last unmentionable taboo: menstruation' and the surprisingly long-lasting theme of 'feminine hygeine'. American.

WEBSITES

If you know you have a specific condition, use your search engine to search for websites using key words. If you don't have access to the World Wide Web through a home computer, try your local library or internet café. (If you turn off the picture function, the downloading of words from a website will speed up and therefore be cheaper.)

www.awhn.org.au/home.htm
The Australian Women's Health Network
Women's health advocacy network run by volunteers which lobby the government and try to post important and useful links and information on many women's health subjects. Go to the Women's Health Issues link on their home page and click on your area of interest.

SUPPORT GROUPS

The following contact points can be used to find specific support groups for your illness, information and advice and for various contacts in your area. These groups nearly always have their funding cut, so you can help out by ringing your local politician to say we need them properly funded.

Women's Information Services
These groups will be able to point you in any direction you need. They're a clearing house for any requests for information.

Australian Capital Territory
Women's Information Referral Centre
Level 6, 197 London Circuit
Canberra City ACT 2600
Phone: 02 6205 1075, 02 6205 1076
Fax: 02 6205 1077
Email: wirc@act.gov.au
Homepage: www.act.gov.au

New South Wales
Women's Information and Referral Service
Department for Women
Level 4, 181 Castlereagh Street
Sydney NSW 2000
Phone: 02 9287 1810, 1800 817 227
Fax: 02 9287 1823
Email: dfw@women.nsw.gov.au
Homepage: www.women.nsw.gov.au

Northern Territory

Darwin
Women's Health Strategy Unit
PO Box 40 596
Casuarina NT 0811
Phone: 08 8999 2804

Alice Springs
Women's Information Centre
Ground floor, Eurilpa House, Todd Mall
Alice Springs NT 0870
PO Box 721, Alice Springs NT 0871
Phone: 08 8951 5880
Fax: 08 8951 5884
Email: wicalice.ths@nt.gov.au

Queensland
Brisbane
Women's Information Link
56 Mary Street
Brisbane QLD 4000
PO Box 185, Albert Street
Brisbane QLD 4002
Phone: 07 3224 2211, 1800 177 577
Fax: 1800 656 122
Email: infolink@premiers.qld.gov.au
Homepage: www.qldwoman.qld.gov.au

Cairns
Women's Information and Referral Centre
230 Mulgrave Street
Cairns QLD 4870
Phone: 07 4051 9366
Fax: 07 4031 6750
Email: wirc@wirc.org.au

South Australia
Women's Information Service
136 North Terrace, Station Arcade
Adelaide SA 5000
Phone: 08 8303 0590, 1800 188 158
Fax: 08 8303 0576
Email: info@wif.sa.gov.au
Homepage: www.wif.sa.gov.au

Tasmania
Women Tasmania
140–142 Macquarie Street
Hobart TAS 7000
Phone: 03 6233 2208, 1800 001 377
Fax: 03 6233 8833
Email: wt.admin@dpac.tas.gov.au
Homepage: www.women.tas.gov.au

Victoria
Women's Information and Referral Exchange
1st floor, 247 Flinders Lane
Melbourne VIC 3000

Phone: 03 9206 0870, 1300 134 130
Fax: 03 9654 6831
Email: wire@wire.org.au
Homepage: www.wire@org.au

Western Australia
Women's Information Service
1st floor, 141 St George's Terrace
Perth WA 6000
Phone: 08 9264 1900, 1800 199 174
Fax: 08 9264 1925
Email: wpo@fcs.wa.gov.au
Homepage: www.wa.gov.au/wpdo

Family Planning Clinics
For information on general women's health and screening matters as well as contraception and pregnancy termination, you can't go past the Family Planning Clinics. Here are their head offices. Phone for a service nearer you.

Australian Capital Territory
Health Promotion Centre
Childers Street
Canberra ACT 2600
GPO Box 1317, Canberra City ACT 2601
Phone: 02 6247 3077
Fax: 02 6257 5710
Email: fpact@familyplanningact.org.au
Homepage: www.familyplanningact.org

New South Wales
FPA Health
328–336 Liverpool Road
Ashfield NSW 2131
Phone: 02 8752 4300, 1300 658 886
Fax: 02 9716 6164
Email: enquiries@fpahealth.org.au
Homepage: www.fpahealth.org.au

Northern Territory
Family Planning Welfare
The Clock Tower, Unit 2
Dickward Drive
Coconut Grove NT 0810
Phone: 08 8948 1044
Fax: 08 8948 0626

Queensland
Family Planning Queensland (FPQ)
100 Alfred Street
Fortitude Valley QLD 4006
Phone: 07 3250 0200
Fax: 07 3854 1277
Homepage: www.fpq.asn.au

South Australia
Shine SA
17 Phillips Street
Kensington SA 5068

Phone: 08 8431 5177, 1800 188 171
Fax: 08 8364 2389
Homepage: www.shinesa.org.au

Tasmania
Family Planning Tasmania Inc.
2 Midwood Street
New Town TAS 7008
Phone: 03 6228 5244, 1800 007 119
Email: FamPlan.Hobt@tassie.net.au
Homepage: www.tased.edu.au/tasonline/scxedfpt

Victoria
Family Planning Victoria
901 Whitehorse Road
Box Hill VIC 3128
Phone: 03 9257 0100, 1800 013 952
Fax: 03 9257 0112
Email: fpv@fpv.org.au
Homepage: www.sexlife.com

Western Australia
Family Planning Western Australia
70 Roe Street
Northbridge WA 6003
Phone: 08 9227 6177, 1800 198 205
Fax: 08 9227 6871
Email: sexhelp@fpwa-health.org.au
Homepage: www.fpwa-health.org.au

HEALTH CARE CENTRES

For help in locating services and finding support groups
and information about medical conditions. Call the relevant numbers to find local contacts in your suburb,
district or town.

Australian Capital Territory
Women's Health Service
Corner Moore and Alinga Streets
Canberra City ACT 2601
Phone: 02 6205 1078
Fax: 02 6207 0143

New South Wales
Women's Medical Centre
Suite 10 and 11, level 2
193 Macquarie Street
Sydney NSW 2000
Phone: 02 9231 2366
Fax: 02 9233 1020
Homepage: www.womensmedicalcentre.com

Northern Territory
Royal Darwin Hospital
Rockland Drive
Tiwi NT 0810
Phone: 08 8922 8888
Fax: 08 8922 8286
Homepage:
www.nt.gov.au/nths/royaldarwinhospital/welcome.htm

Queensland
Women's Health Queensland Wide
165 Gregory Terrace
Springhill QLD 4000
Phone: 07 3839 9962, 1800 017 676
Fax: 07 3831 7214
Email: whcb@womhealth.org.au
Homepage: www.womhealth.org.au

South Australia
Women's Health Statewide
64 Pennington Terrace
North Adelaide SA 5006
Phone: 08 8239 9600, 1800 182 098
Fax: 08 8239 9696
Email: info@whs.sa.gov.au
Homepage: www.whs.sa.gov.au

Tasmania
Hobart Women's Health Centre
326 Elizabeth Street
North Hobart TAS 7000
Phone: 03 6231 3212, 1800 353 212
Fax: 03 6236 9449
Email: hwhc@trump.net.au
Homepage: www.tased.edu.au/tasonline/hwhc/hwhc.htm

Victoria
Women's Health Victoria
Level 1, 123 Lonsdale Street
Melbourne VIC 3000
GPO Box 1160K, Melbourne VIC 3001
Phone: 03 9662 3755
Fax: 03 9663 7955
Health information line: 03 9662 3742, 1800 133 321
Email: whv@whv.org.au
Homepage: www.whv.org.au

Western Australia
Women's Health Care House
100 Aberdeen Street
Northbridge WA 6003
Phone: 08 9227 8122, 1800 998 399
Fax: 08 9227 6615
Email: whch@iinet.net.au
Homepage: www.womenshealthwa.iinet.net.au

Index

blood sugar abnormalities
   functional hypoglycaemia 64, 69,
      183–9
   insulin resistance 121–2, 131,
      189–91
blood tests for pregnancy 9, 140
BMI calculation 51–2
body-fat composition 37
bone density 10
   and dieting 47
   magnesium for 252–3
   and overexercising 57
   phyto-oestrogens for 199
books on period problems 258–9
breast cancer 20, 28, 35
breast-feeding and stopped periods
   117
breasts
   checks 138–9, 224
   development of 19, 115–16
   in pregnancy 18, 23
   soreness 205

caffeine intake 60, 97, 244
calcium
   and dieting 47, 49
   low-kilojoule sources 255
   recommended daily allowance
      254–5
   sources 256–7
   supplements 59
carbohydrate-restricted diets 50
carbohydrates 194
   combining 230
   copmplex 229–30
carrier proteins 25
cervical abnormalities 103–4
cervical cancer 103–4
cervical dysplasia 103–4
cervical ectropion 103
cervical eversion 103
cervicitis 104
check-ups 224–5

chemicals, exposure to 22–3
chicken broth 172
chiropractic 87, 182
chloasma 142
cholesterol 16, 233
cigarette smoking 37, 61
cleansing diets 48–9
cocaine 61
coffee 60, 97, 244
cold-pressed oils 237
colposcopy 138
complex carbohydrates 229–30
condoms 10
congestive dysmenorrhoea 79, 86
constipation
   before period 80
   natural therapy for 86
contraceptives 9, 10, 93
corpus luteum 6–7, 24
   insufficiency 39
corticosteroids 24
counting the days 4–5
cramping pain 13, 14, 27, 78–80

D&C (dilatation and curettage) 160
dairy products 237–8
detox diets 47, 48–9
diarrhoea 78
diet 10, 32
   high fibre 50
   high-protein low-carbohydrate
      50
   therapeutic 228, 231
   see also healthy eating, hints for
diet pills 54
dieting
   and bone density 47
   effects on period 47–50
   self care 50–1
diuretics 154, 221–3
doctor, choosing 133–5
dopamine 17

273

275